Hypertension in the Older Adult

Edited by ANDREW K SCOTT MB ChB MD FRCP ——————————

Senior Lecturer and Honorary Consultant in Geriatric Medicine at the University of
Manchester and Salford Royal Hospitals NHS Trust

A member of the Hodder Headline Group
LONDON • SYDNEY • AUCKLAND
Co-published in the USA by
Oxford University Press, Inc., New York

This book is dedicated to my late wife Dorothy,
without whose constant support and encouragement, it would never have
seen the light of day

First published in Great Britain in 1997 by
Arnold, a member of the Hodder Headline Group,
338 Euston Road, London NW1 3BH

Co-published in the United States of America by
Oxford University Press, Inc.,
198 Madison Avenue, New York, NY10016
Oxford is a registered trademark of Oxford University Press

British Library Cataloguing in Publication Data
A catalogue record for this book is available from the British Library

Library of Congress Cataloging-in-Publication Data
A catalog record for this book is available from the Library of Congress

ISBN 0 340 614757

Composition in 10/11 Times and Optima by Phoenix Photosetting, Chatham, Kent
Printed in Great Britain by J W Arrowsmith Ltd, Bristol
Bound by Bookcraft (Bath) Ltd, Midsomer Norton, Bath

Contents

List of contributors   iv
Preface   v

1. **Introduction**   *A K Scott*   1

2. **Epidemiology of blood pressure in the older adult**   *A Fletcher*   6

3. **Pathogenesis of hypertension**   *R D N Tunbridge*   21

4. **Benefits of treatment**   *A K Scott*   39

5. **Clinical pharmacology of antihypertensive drugs in the older adult**
    J Webster   68

6. **Ambulatory blood pressure in the older adult and blood pressure
    measurement**   *J Duggan and E O'Brien*   103

7. **Non-pharmacological treatments for hypertension in the older adult**
    P R Jackson, W W Yeo and L E Ramsay   129

8. **Cost-effectiveness of treating hypertension in the older adult**
    D Coyle   148

9. **The effects of antihypertensive therapy on psychomotor
    performance, quality of life, symptoms and laboratory
    parameters**   *D R Lee and S H D Jackson*   161

10. **Overview**   *A K Scott*   184

Appendix   197
Index   198

List of Contributors

Eoin O'Brien MD, FRCP(Lond), FRCP (Edin), FRCP (Irel)
Professor of Cardiovascular Medicine, Director, Blood Pressure Unit, Beaumont
Hospital, Dublin, Ireland

Douglas Coyle MA, MSc
Lecturer, Faculty of Medicine, University of Ottawa, and Health Economist,
Clinical Epidemiology Unit, Ottawa Civic Hospital, Ontario, Canada

Joe Duggan MD, FRCPI
Consultant Physician and Geriatrician, Department Of Medicine for the Elderly,
James Connolly Memorial Mater and Beaumont Hospital, Dublin, Ireland

Astrid E Fletcher PhD
Reader in Epidemiology, Department of Epidemiology and Population Sciences,
London School of Hygiene and Tropical Medicine, London, United Kingdom

Peter R Jackson MD, ChB, PhD, FRCP
Senior Lecturer in Clinical Pharmacology and Therapeutics, University
Department of Medicine and Pharmacology, Royal Hallamshire Hospital,
Sheffield, United Kingdom

Stephen HD Jackson MD, FRCP
Professor, Department of Health Care of the Elderly, King's College School of
Medicine and Dentistry, Denmark Hill, London, United Kingdom

Dan R Lee MB, BCh, MRCP
Senior Registrar in Medicine for Elderly People, Whipps Cross Hospital,
Leytonstone, London, United Kingdom

Lawrence E Ramsay MB, ChB, FRCP
Professor of Clinical Pharmacology and Therapeutics, University Department of
Medicine and Pharmacology, Royal Hallamshire Hospital, Sheffield, United
Kingdom

Andrew K Scott B.Med.Biol; MB, ChB, MD, FRCP
Senior Lecturer and Honorary Consultant, Department of Geriatric Medicine,
Hope Hospital, Manchester, United Kingdom

David Tunbridge MD, FRCP
Senior Lecturer in Medicine, Department of Medicine, Manchester Royal
Infirmary, United Kingdom

John Webster MD, FRCP(Edin)
Consultant Physician, Aberdeen Royal Infirmary, United Kingdom

Wilfred W Yeo MB, ChB, MD, MRCP
Lecturer in Clinical Pharmacology and Therapeutics, University Department of
Medicine and Pharmacology, Royal Hallamshire Hospital, Sheffield, United
Kingdom

Preface

Heart disease and stroke are by far the most important causes of death in older adults. There is as yet no effective treatment for acute stroke and therapy is aimed at limiting disability. While thrombolytic agents and aspirin have improved the outcome in acute myocardial infarction there is still considerable morbidity and mortality. The prognosis for those patients who develop cardiac failure is worse than for many malignant tumours.

Preventing or delaying the onset of such vascular diseases must be the main target of any health service. Hypertension is the single most important risk factor that is amenable to treatment and which has an extensive body of evidence to show that treatment is effective. Older patients are at greater risk of a vascular event than younger patients for the same level of blood pressure. They have much to gain from successful treatment of hypertension in a holistic setting that treats the blood pressure and other important risk factors for the individual patient.

Interest in treating hypertension in older adults has been increasing over the last 10–15 years. This is reflected in a rapidly expanding literature on all aspects of hypertension in this age group. Since hypertension is a common disorder and the elderly population continues to increase there is a need for all health professionals to be aware of its diagnosis and management. At the time this volume was conceived, there was no text dealing exclusively with hypertension in elderly patients.

The aim of this book is to provide comprehensive coverage of all aspects of hypertension in older adults with a view to improving management of hypertension in the section of the population at greatest risk from it. We also aim to contribute to the debate about controversial issues, encourage attention to the sometimes less palatable economic issues, and finally, hope to stimulate further research in areas that have received little coverage.

Andrew K Scott
1997

CHAPTER 1

Introduction

ANDREW K SCOTT ———————————————————————

Elderly patients have often been excluded from clinical trials, even in conditions that predominantly affect this age group. Treatment of many diseases in the elderly is thus often difficult to justify in scientific terms because of the lack of good quality clinical trials that have included adequate numbers of older subjects. Even when elderly patients are included in studies of illness with a high prevalence in older adults there is a tendency for the younger elderly patients to be over-represented with relatively low numbers of patients over the age of 80. Our relative ignorance about the 'old elderly' is a matter for concern, as they are the group which will undergo the most rapid expansion in the coming decades.

Hypertension is a common problem in elderly patients and is one of the few conditions in which the evidence of benefit from treatment is actually stronger than in younger adults. However, hypertension trials published to date have failed to address the problem of the whole elderly population as noted above. The major outcome trials in elderly hypertensive patients either specifically excluded the very elderly (over age 80 or 84) or recruited too few very elderly patients to allow a clear answer on the benefits of treatment.

In historical terms, the treatment of hypertension in elderly patients is very recent with treatment of the over 70 age group being a reasonably common practice only in the past 10 years. Many of the pioneers of cardiovascular research and measurement of blood pressure exceeded their three score years and ten – William Harvey, discoverer of the circulation of the blood, lived to be 78; Reverend Stephen Hales (83) measured arterial pressure in a horse; Sir William Withey Gull (74) demonstrated thickening of the walls of smaller arteries. Such distinguished scientists would have been unable to measure blood pressure in humans and would of course have been unable to treat it whatever their age. Reliable blood pressure measurement has been available for almost a century but well tolerated antihypertensive drugs have been around for less than 50 years. Initial trials understandably concentrated on younger adults but as the age for inclusion increased in some of the studies, it tended to stick at 69 with 'elderly' being regarded as age 60–69 years. This resulted in considerable debate as to whether or not to treat older patients. Even today we are still uncertain as to whether the very elderly (over 85 years) should be treated. Fortunately there is now increasing interest in the health needs of elderly people with more emphasis on all aspects of clinical and basic research into the problems of old age. Research into hypertension in the elderly is one of the growth areas.

In discussing hypertension in elderly patients we first need to consider what we mean by hypertension and what we mean by elderly. It has long been known that blood pressure changes with age and this is covered in Chapter 2. Traditionally, the threshold for treating hypertension in older adults has been higher at around 160/100 mmHg than in younger adults where 140/90 mmHg is often quoted. This has occurred despite the epidemiological evidence that for any level of blood pressure the risks of a cardiovascular event are greater in older patients. Even the results of recent studies showing greater benefit in terms of number of patient-years of treatment necessary to prevent one cardiovascular event have not really changed standard thinking on these values. The level above which elderly patients should be treated seems about right and is discussed in Chapter 4. However, is it really justified to treat many hundreds of younger patients with relatively low levels of blood pressure to prevent one event? Where should the line be drawn? Fortunately we do not have to address this very difficult question in the present book, which is focused on the elderly.

What do we mean by 'elderly'? Old age is usually taken as the age at which we retire or become eligible for our old-age pension. However, this figure is an arbitrary one originally introduced by Bismarck in 1873. It has more to do with allowing turnover in the job-market and giving a reasonable sized retired population that can be supported by the state, than any medical definition of old. That is to say, it is a social construct rather than a biological fact. Attitudes of older people are changing, with most living an active and healthy life for many years into retirement. Many older people do not consider themselves elderly at 70 or even 75. Many geriatricians run a service that is at least partly age related. The cut-off age is as low as 65 in some centres but a more usual cut-off is between 75 and 80 years. This raises the question as to what is the best cut-off age to determine that a patient with hypertension is allocated to the elderly group. A pragmatic approach seems reasonable. The early studies of hypertension in older patients took 60 years as the minimum age of entry and much evidence is based on this figure. For the purposes of this book, we have accepted 60 years as the definition of elderly.

The pathological changes and complications of hypertension are common in elderly people. These are discussed in Chapter 3. Few of the observed pathological changes and none of the complications are exclusive to patients with hypertension. Stroke and myocardial infarction are common in the elderly population even with normal blood pressure. The cardiovascular diseases we are trying to prevent have many risk factors and these require attention in a holistic, or at least multifactorial, approach to patient management. Some aspects of this are discussed in Chapter 7. Many doctors have been too ready to accept that merely treating blood pressure with any antihypertensive agents will result in a reduction in complications from hypertension. Others have been reluctant to act on the results of the good quality, multicentre trials which have shown benefit in treating elderly hypertensive patients and have been slow to treat their patients. The evidence for treating hypertension in elderly patients is discussed in Chapter 4, although there is still much to be done before we have a clear answer as to whether or not all antihypertensive drugs produce benefits in elderly patients with mild/moderate hypertension. In addition, we require studies to show which drugs work best in combination in terms of preventing complications. Studies published to date have had too few patients on combined treatment to show clearly whether two drugs are better than one. There are no studies comparing different second-line drugs when added to the first-choice agent.

When drugs are used in elderly patients we need to consider the effect age and (since multiple pathology is common) concurrent disease have on both pharmacokinetics and pharmacodynamics. This is particularly important when selecting agents from within a group that contains drugs with a variety of properties such as different routes of elimination, different half-life times and duration of effect, and different adverse effects that might be a particular problem in older patients. Such factors are discussed in Chapter 5.

Hypertension is often considered to be easy to diagnose. However, setting aside the debate over the level at which treatment should be started, there are still major problems in the way the diagnosis is made. The multicentre studies showed that many patients (up to 50%!) achieved normal blood pressure on treatment with placebo. These patients clearly do not have sustained hypertension, but are they at increased risk of cardiovascular events? There is little evidence to support the need for treatment in this group or to show that they do not benefit from treatment. If diagnosis of sustained hypertension is poor in the clinical trial situation, it is likely to be much worse in routine practice. In addition, there are the well-known problems of poor maintenance of equipment even in hospitals (Conceico *et al.*, 1979; Shaw *et al.*, 1979), poor technique of measurement by both doctors and nurses and ignorance of the many factors that need to be controlled while measuring blood pressure. The flat blood pressure chart with constant systolic and diastolic pressures over a period of time is still a common occurrence and many junior doctors do not measure blood pressure themselves but simply take the reading from the nursing chart. Do senior doctors without an interest in hypertension ever check the blood pressure themselves on a ward round? Disquiet with performance at measuring blood pressure and difficulty in making a diagnosis of sustained hypertension with a standard clinic technique has understandably led to research into other methods of diagnosis. Ambulatory blood pressure monitoring has been intensively studied in younger adults and is being increasingly used in older patients both for research and to a lesser extent in routine practice. This is discussed in Chapter 6.

Many elderly patients prefer not to take medication and are enthusiastic about lifestyle changes and non-pharmacological measures that can lower the blood pressure. Others of course can't or won't alter their lifelong habits. However, when the patient is willing to use non-drug methods of lowering blood pressure these may, in addition, reduce other cardiovascular risk factors and bring other health benefits. These are reviewed in Chapter 7. Unfortunately we have no evidence of benefit in terms of reduced morbidity and mortality from such forms of treatment but this may be available in the near future.

Costs of treatment are becoming increasingly important for all health care delivery systems, irrespective of whether they are funded privately or out of the public purse. All health care systems have limited funding and are looking for ways to contain costs. Since hypertension is a common condition, the costs of treating it will have a major influence on the overall health budget. The cost clearly needs to be offset against the benefits of treatment and the cost-benefits of hypertension treatment are considered in Chapter 8. One difficulty in making cost comparisons is that doctors in routine practice don't always prescribe in the ways suggested by clinical trials. This can have a significant effect on overall costs and result in a different best buy from that predicted from clinical trials.

Patients with hypertension are generally well with no symptoms due to their hypertension. It has been clearly shown in younger age groups that just labelling someone as 'hypertensive' increases the amount of 'illness' they experience and time spent off work (Haynes *et al.*, 1978; Polk *et al.*, 1984; Wagner and Stogatz, 1985). In addition, no drug is completely free from adverse effects and some of these are intolerable. It is difficult to persuade patients to take medication if they feel the drug is causing problems and in some cases, all drugs seem to cause difficulties. Quality of life is very important. This needs to be made a high priority so that treatment does not just add years to life but ensures that those years are enjoyable. Adverse effects and quality of life are discussed in Chapter 9. The frequency of adverse effects may differ in older patients compared with younger adults, and some adverse effects of antihypertensives seem particularly troublesome in the elderly; for example leg oedema with the dihydropyridine calcium channel blockers. Greater care needs to be taken with drug selection for individual patients to ensure a good quality of life while minimising their risk of stroke or myocardial infarction.

When this volume was conceived there was no textbook dealing exclusively with hypertension in elderly patients. Several reviews had been published and increasing interest was being shown in performing studies of all aspects of hypertension in elderly patients. Hypertension in older adults is very important, since it is more common in this age group and each individual patient is at higher risk of developing a disease event due to the hypertension. It was felt therefore that there was a need for a book to bring together all of the information relevant to hypertension in the elderly. The aim of the book is to review and summarise all aspects of hypertension from epidemiology through pathogenesis, diagnosis, treatment, economics and quality of life, using data from studies in older patients wherever possible. It was accepted that in some situations there would be no data from elderly subjects and the results from younger adults would need to be used, with discussion of how these might apply to older age groups and whether further research is necessary. Each chapter has been written so that it can be read without excessive reference to other sections. A small amount of overlap has therefore been included. The book is written to appeal to everyone involved in the management of elderly patients with hypertension.

The risk with all textbooks is that they rapidly become out of date. This is particularly relevant with hypertension in the elderly as several important outcome trials are ongoing and should be reporting within the next few years. Important trials published up to the last possible moment have been included. The next 10 years promise to be an exciting time for those involved in treating hypertension in older patients as more is found out about diagnosis and cost-effective treatment, and, more particularly, when definitive evidence is obtained on which groups of drugs are most effective for preventing both cardiac and cerebrovascular complications.

REFERENCES

Conceico S, Ward MK, Kerr DNS 1979. Defects in sphygmomanometers: an important source of error in blood pressure recording. *British Medical Journal* **1**, 886–8.

Haynes RB, Sackett DL, Taylor DW, Gibson ES, Johnson AL 1978. Increased absenteeism from work after detection and labelling of hypertensive patients. *New England Journal of Medicine* **299**, 741–4.

Polk BF, Harlan LC, Copper SP *et al.* 1984. Disability days associated with detection and treatment in a hypertension control program. *American Journal of Epidemiology* **119**, 44–53.

Shaw A, Deehan C, Lenihan JMA 1979. Sphygmomanometers: errors due to blocked vents. *British Medical Journal* **1**, 789–90.

Wagner EH, Stogatz DS 1985. Hypertension labelling and well-being: alternative explanations in cross sectional data. *Journal of Chronic Disease* **38**, 37–45.

CHAPTER 2

Epidemiology of blood pressure in the older adult

ASTRID FLETCHER

THE DISTRIBUTION OF BLOOD PRESSURE WITH AGE

The relationship between blood pressure and age has been described for many populations, predominantly in developed countries. The data have been derived primarily from cross-sectional studies but there are also a few longitudinal studies. The results are well illustrated by recent data from the Health Survey for England (OPCS, 1994) (Fig. 2.1a and b). Fig. 2.1a shows an association between increasing age and increasing systolic blood pressure, both in men and in women; for diastolic pressure an association with increasing age is observed until middle age (50–60 years), but thereafter plateaus, with some suggestion in men of a fall in the very elderly (age 75 years) (Fig. 2.1b). Cross-sectional analyses need to be interpreted with caution since the relationship of blood pressure to age may reflect blood pressure differences between different birth cohorts rather than age-related changes in blood pressure. However, almost identical findings have been observed in longitudinal analyses, such as of the Framingham study, where a cohort has been followed over time (Kannel and Gordon, 1978).

It has been noted that these relationships between age and blood pressure are remarkably consistent across North American, European and Japanese populations as well as in some developing countries, although the average values of blood pressures between populations differ (Whelton *et al.*, 1994). Differences between men and women in mean blood pressure levels and the rate of rise of blood pressure also show some consistency across populations. In nearly all developed countries, young adult women have lower systolic and diastolic pressures than men. However, the rate of rise of blood pressure with age is steeper for women from around the menopause, especially for systolic pressure, and in many populations women have higher systolic blood pressures than men by the sixth and seventh decades. In the Health Survey of England, between the ages of 35 to 44 years, systolic blood pressure in men was an average 9 mmHg higher than in women (135 mmHg in men and 126 mmHg in women). By middle age (55–64 years), this difference was attenuated to a 2 mmHg difference (146 mmHg in men and 144 mmHg in women) and by the sixth and seventh

(a)

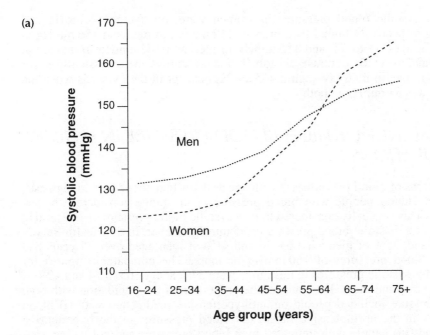

(b)

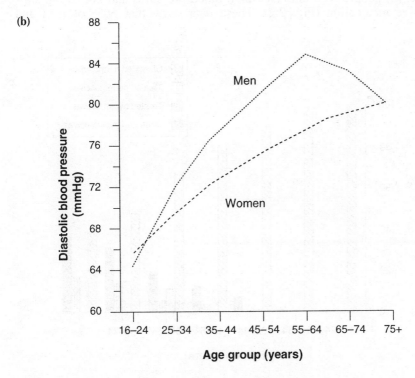

Fig. 2.1 (a) Systolic blood pressure by age. (b) Diastolic blood pressure by age

decades, systolic blood pressures in women were, on average 4 mmHg and 7 mmHg respectively higher than in men (152 mmHg in men and 156 mmHg in women at ages 65 to 74, and 155 mmHg in men and 162 mmHg in women at ages 75 and over). By contrast, diastolic blood pressures were consistently lower in women than in men (averaging 4–5 mmHg) except in the over 75s when the average was 81 mmHg in both.

PREVALENCE OF HIGH BLOOD PRESSURE IN ELDERLY POPULATIONS

The patterns of blood pressure rise with age as described above lead to high estimates of elderly people with blood pressure in the range considered 'hypertensive'. This is usually considered to be a systolic blood pressure of 160 mmHg or over, or a diastolic blood pressure of 95 mmHg or over. In the Health Survey for England, 35% of men aged 65–74 and 41% of men aged over 75 years had systolic blood pressures of 160 mmHg or more. The comparable figures for women for systolic pressures in this range were 37% at ages 65 to 74 and 49% at ages 75 years and more. Estimates of the proportion of the population with high blood pressure included people on antihypertensive medication with (i) blood pressures in the normotensive range, (ii) blood pressures in the hypertensive range and (iii) people with untreated high blood pressures and not taking antihypertensive medication (Fig. 2.2). These data show that 50% of men and

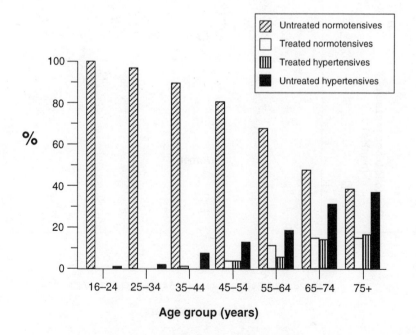

Fig. 2.2   Classes of hypertensives and normotensives by age

women aged 65 to 74 years were classified as having high blood pressure. Of these 13% were treated normotensives, 12% had high blood pressures despite treatment, and 26% had untreated high blood pressure. The proportions were relatively similar for men and women in this age group. Proportions for the over 75 age group showed 56% of men and 70% of women categorised as having high blood pressure, most of the excess in women being accounted for by a higher proportion of hypertensive women on antihypertensive medication with blood pressures still in the hypertensive range. It is likely that in these, as in many other blood pressure survey data, the estimates both of average blood pressure levels and proportion with hypertension based on a single visit are likely to be over-estimated. Regression to the mean, white-coat hypertension, and increased variability of blood pressure (especially in old age) (Veerman *et al.*, 1994) usually result in higher blood pressures at the first screen (even when several blood pressure readings are taken). Several studies have shown that the prevalence of sustained hypertension, i.e. consistently high levels of blood pressure measured over several occasions, is about one third of that for casual measurements (Colandrea *et al.*, 1970; Miall and Greenberg, 1987). Blood pressure measurement in the elderly is associated with more sources of error than in younger age groups. The increased rigidity of the arterial wall may lead to over-estimation of blood pressure, while a large auscultatory gap is likely to result in an under-estimation of systolic blood pressure (Swales, 1995). Elderly people also demonstrate quite substantial post-prandial falls in blood pressure and therefore blood pressure measurements taken within 2 hours of a meal will lead to an under-estimate of the usual blood pressure (Macrae and Bulpitt, 1989). Seasonal variation in blood pressure is also heightened in older adults. Woodhouse and colleagues (1993) found a fourfold increase in the proportion of elderly subjects (aged 65 to 74 years) with blood pressures over 160/90 mmHg in winter compared with summer.

Ambulatory blood pressure measurements over a 24-hour period avoid some of the problems of the elevated pressure seen with a single clinic visit. Studies consistently show lower blood pressures based on ambulatory readings compared with clinic readings (O'Brien *et al.*, 1991). The prediction of cardiovascular risk from ambulatory blood pressures is not yet known, although this question is being examined in one large prospective study (Amery *et al.*, 1991). Until these data are available it would be unwise to base treatment decisions only on ambulatory blood pressure levels.

In recent years there has been more emphasis on the importance of 'isolated systolic hypertension' (ISH), i.e. a high systolic blood pressure but proportionately lower diastolic pressure, usually defined as a systolic blood pressure of 160 mmHg or more, and a diastolic pressure less than 95 or 90 mmHg. As might be expected from the age-related changes described above, isolated systolic hypertension is common in elderly people and continues to rise into extremes of old age (Fig. 2.1a and b). In a meta-analysis of population studies of ISH, the pooled estimates of prevalence of isolated systolic hypertension was 0.1% at 40 years, 0.8% at 50 years, 5% at 60 years, 12.6% at 70 years and 23.6% at 80 years (Staessen *et al.*, 1990b). However these figures were mostly based on casual measurements of blood pressure and sustained isolated systolic hypertension prevalence is likely to be lower. On average the prevalence was 43% higher in women than in men. A higher prevalence was also found in patients on antihypertensive medication, suggesting that treatment was more effective in controlling the diastolic pressures. However, inadequate management may also be an explanation. Blood pressure goals for hypertensive patients, especially elderly patients, until relatively recently, emphasise the diastolic pressures with goal blood pressures frequently being only just below the target threshold for treatment. Some evidence for a proportion of ISH reflecting poor management is provided by the Systolic Hypertension in the Elderly Program (SHEP) in which around one third of the patients who were entered into the trial had previously uncontrolled ISH on treatment. Average blood pressure reductions in the trial were 26 mmHg systolic and 9 mmHg diastolic, which were associated with a 36% reduction in stroke and 27% reduction in coronary heart disease (CHD) (SHEP Co-operative Research Group, 1991). These reductions were of a similar magnitude in actively treated patients irrespective of previous antihypertensive treatment. Thus it can be concluded from the SHEP study that a more proactive treatment policy of previously treated patients with ISH resulted in blood pressure falls and hence less cardiovascular disease.

Postural orthostatic hypotension (OH) also occurs more frequently in elderly people. Prevalence estimates of orthostatic hypotension vary widely with the definition, and characteristics of the population, in particular with the age range and health status (Rutan *et al.*, 1992). A usual definition of OH is a fall of 20 mmHg or more in systolic blood pressure or 10 mmHg or more in diastolic blood pressure, from the supine blood pressure to the standing blood pressure measured after standing for 3 minutes. Prevalence rates of 16% were found in one study of people aged 65 years and over but only 2% were symptomatic. Major ECG abnormalities and carotid artery stenosis and a decreased body-mass index (BMI) were associated with OH. In the SHEP trial the prevalence of OH (based on the systolic blood pressure only) was 10% but only 3% of these reported troublesome dizziness (a similar proportion to participants without OH); OH was associated with higher systolic blood pressures and lower BMIs but not with any markers of cardiovascular disease (Applegate *et al.*, 1991). Whether OH independently increases mortality risk (other than by its association with increased numbers of falls) has yet to be demonstrated.

BLOOD PRESSURE TRACKING

Blood pressure tracking refers to the observation that the rate of rise of blood pressure with age is strongly influenced by the initial blood pressure level; thus subjects in the highest percentile of blood pressure in early adult life have the greatest increase in blood pressure in later life (Miall and Lovell, 1967; Svardsudd and Tibblin, 1980). The relative contributions of genetic influences and environmental risk factors to tracking are not understood. In recent years the work of Barker and colleagues (1989) has suggested that factors operating in the foetal environment predict subsequent cardiovascular outcomes. A strong inverse relationship was also found between birth weight, and the ratio of placental weight to birth weight, and blood pressure levels in middle age (Law and Barker, 1994).

DETERMINANTS OF HIGH BLOOD PRESSURE IN ELDERLY PEOPLE

The notion that the rise in blood pressure was an inevitable consequence of physiological changes associated with ageing was challenged by studies which showed that, for example, in some rural communities in developing countries, there was no evidence for a rise in blood pressure across adult life (Epstein and Eckoff, 1967; Poulter *et al.*, 1985; Shaper, 1967). These populations were typically low blood pressure populations, often geographically and culturally isolated. Several studies have shown that when individuals from such populations migrate to urbanised environments, blood pressures rise shortly after migration (Poulter *et al.*, 1990). It seems likely that the rise in blood pressure with age is, in part, explained by the determinants of blood pressure.

Sodium intake

Evidence for a relationship between sodium and blood pressure has been provided by studies between populations, within populations and from randomised trials of sodium reduction. There is general agreement that sodium influences blood pressure, but less agreement on the magnitude of the relationship from individual studies. Problems in the accurate estimation of sodium from a single 24-hour measurement means that estimates of effect are likely to be underestimated (regression dilution bias). Several studies and pooled overviews of data have estimated an effect of an increase of 4–5 mmHg systolic and 2 mmHg diastolic for every 100 mmol increase of sodium in both between population and within population studies (Elliott, 1991; Law *et al.*, 1991a, 1991b).

The effect of sodium on blood pressure increases with age and with level of blood pressure, for example, at ages 60–69 years an increase of 100 mmol of sodium is associated with a 10 mmHg rise in systolic blood pressure, and for persons of this age on the 95th centile of the blood pressure distribution a 15 mmHg increase in systolic blood pressure (Law *et al.*, 1991a). This increased relationship of sodium and blood pressure with age may reflect the adverse effects on blood pressure of lifetime exposure to sodium or age related changes in the ability to maintain sodium balance.

Increase in weight

Cross-sectional studies have shown a strong relationship between body weight and blood pressure at all ages (Chiang *et al.*, 1969; Dyer and Elliot, 1989; Stamler *et al.*, 1978). In the Health Survey for England a stepwise increase in the proportion with high blood pressure with increasing BMI was observed (Fig. 2.3a and b). Nearly 70% of men and 80% of women aged over 65 years who were in the highest BMI level (BMI over 30) had high blood pressure. Around 12% of men over 65 years and 18% of women were in this BMI range showing that gross obesity in elderly people is not uncommon and is an important health problem. The INTERSALT study found that for a given average height, a 10 kg difference in body weight was associated with a 3 mmHg difference in systolic blood

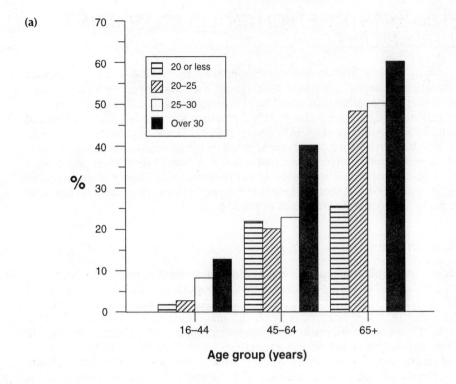

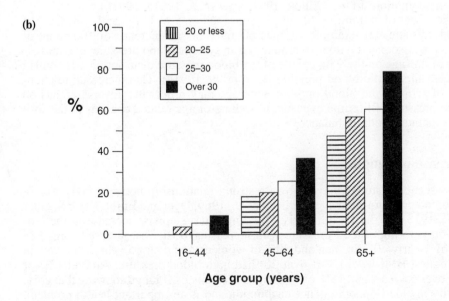

Fig. 2.3 Proportion with high blood pressure by body-mass index and age (a) for men, (b) for women

pressure and a 2.2 mmHg difference in diastolic pressure (Dyer and Elliot, 1989). Body weight in adolescence is a strong predictor of blood pressure in later life, and may in part explain blood pressure tracking (Worynarowska *et al.*, 1985).

Physical exercise

Many observational studies have described an inverse relationship between blood pressure and physical activity or objective measures of physical fitness (Fagard, 1993). The strength and magnitude of the association are difficult to determine from such studies because of possible confounding factors, in particular the self-selection of 'fitter' individuals into the high physical activity groups, and because of considerable variation between studies in the definitions of physical activity. In a follow-up study of college alumni, vigorous exercise was protective against the development of hypertension in later life (Paffenberger *et al.*, 1983). Thus the rise in blood pressure with age may also reflect the effects of a sedentary lifestyle increasing with advancing age.

Studies on the effects of physical exercise training on blood pressure have shown reductions of an average of 10/8 mmHg in hypertensives, 6/7 mmHg in borderline hypertensives, and 3/3 mmHg in normotensives with regimens with a high energy expenditure (Fagard, 1993). The results were independent of age and weight loss.

Alcohol consumption

Many studies have described a relationship between alcohol consumption and blood pressure (World Hypertension League, 1991). In some studies the relationship was linear across the entire range of alcohol consumption, while other studies have suggested a threshold effect of around three units a day. J curves have also been described, perhaps as a result of the inclusion of previously heavy drinkers in the no-drinks group. In the large Kaiser Permanente Study of 80 000 men and women aged 15 to 79 years, systolic pressure increased by 1 mmHg for each daily unit of alcohol (Klatsky *et al.*, 1977). In one US study the rise in blood pressure with alcohol was greater in people aged 50 to 74 years compared with those aged 35 to 49 years (Fortmann *et al.*, 1983). In the Health Survey for England, men who drank more than 35 units of alcohol per week were more likely to have raised blood pressure while, in contrast, men who drank between 1 to 10 units were less likely to have high blood pressure than expected. These findings support to some extent the epidemiological data suggesting that moderate alcohol consumption is protective against cardiovascular disease (Rimm *et al.*, 1991). The pressor effect of alcohol appears to be due to ethanol as it has been found to exist irrespective of whether the alcohol consumed was wine, beer or spirits.

BLOOD PRESSURE AS A CARDIOVASCULAR RISK FACTOR IN ELDERLY PEOPLE

Epidemiologists have advised against undue emphasis on 'hypertension' as a disease and 'normotension' as normal since there is a continuous and positive relationship between blood pressure level in the range 70–110 mmHg and cardiovascular events, including both stroke and coronary heart disease (McMahon *et al.*, 1990). Thus, in most populations with high average blood pressures, all subjects would benefit from a reduction of blood pressure, but the use of pharmacological treatment should depend on the level of risk and the consequent ratio of costs and benefits. The elderly with hypertension are examples of such high-risk groups, but treatment decisions still need to take into account the absolute level of risk in a particular country and the relative proportions of CHD and stroke events.

Although most of this data is based on middle-aged subjects, studies such as the Framingham study have confirmed the prognostic significance of a raised blood pressure in subjects principally in the age range 65–74 years (Harris *et al.*, 1988). The risk of isolated systolic hypertension is also well established, based on data from middle-aged and young-elderly people (Staessen *et al.*, 1990b). In contrast, in the very elderly, studies provide conflicting evidence. An adverse effect of raised blood pressure has been shown in subjects with an average age of 82 years (Aronow *et al.*, 1989), but an inverse relationship between blood pressure level and survival has also been described in studies from Finland (Mattila *et al.*, 1988) and California (Langer *et al.*, 1989) such that those with the lowest pressures had the highest all-cause and cardiovascular mortality. More complex relationships between blood pressure and mortality have been described for the three prospective elderly cohorts in the EPESE study (Established Populations for Epidemiologic Studies of the Elderly; Taylor *et al.*, 1991) and for cohorts in Sweden (Lindholm *et al.*, 1986).

J-shape relationships have also been reported in treated elderly hypertensives (Bulpitt *et al.*, 1992; Cruickshank *et al.*, 1987; Staessen *et al.*, 1989). The relationship is most consistently described for treated diastolic blood pressure and CHD events and is not observed for systolic blood pressure, or for stroke events. It has been suggested that the adverse effect of a treated low diastolic pressure is observed only in ischaemic patients (Cruickshank *et al.*, 1987) but the studies are not consistent in this finding. The main concern is whether the non-linear relationships observed for diastolic pressure and CHD represent a deleterious effect of blood pressure-lowering by drug treatment, or some secondary association reflected by a low blood pressure (Beevers, 1988). The strongest evidence against a treatment-induced causal relationship is the existence of similar relationships both in placebo-treated (European Working Party on Hypertension in the Elderly (EWPHE); Staessen *et al.*, 1989) and untreated patients (Hypertension in Elderly Persons (HEP) trial; Coope and Warrender, 1987) and for non-cardiovascular mortality and treated blood pressure (EWPHE; Staessen *et al.*, 1989).

The HEP trial in the elderly found an increased CHD rate for the lowest diastolic pressures (less than 80 mmHg) in both actively treated patients and the untreated controls with a nadir at 80–90. The EWPHE trial also showed an increased mortality in the lowest strata of the treated diastolic blood pressure distribution. The same phenomenon was observed for patients on placebo, and for non-cardiovascular mortality (Fig. 2.4).

The most common explanation postulated for the loss of a positive association between blood pressure and cardiovascular mortality is the influence of co-morbidity. Thus a low blood pressure may be a consequence of a disease such as

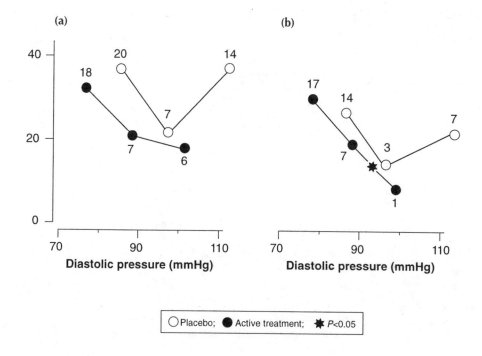

Fig. 2.4 Relationship between diastolic pressure and (a) cardiovascular mortality and (b) non-cardiovascular mortality

cancer or cardiac disease, either through weight loss or some other metabolic disturbance due to the disease. The poor survival is due to the associated co-morbidity rather than the consequential low blood pressure. This explanation would also apply to other chronic vascular disease (CVD) risk factors such as BMI and cholesterol, which also display negative, J- and U-shaped relationships in very elderly people (Fletcher and Bulpitt, 1992; Staessen *et al.*, 1990a).

In a community survey of over 10 000 subjects aged 60 to 79 years death from CHD showed a J-shaped curve with the lowest death rate for an untreated systolic pressure of 160–179 mmHg (Coope *et al.*, 1988). When subjects with cardiac problems, bronchial asthma, diabetes or any serious disease were excluded, the increased mortality at lower pressures effectively disappeared (Fig. 2.5).

The East Boston study of 4000 men and women aged 65 to 79 years described a U-shaped relationship for systolic blood pressure and CVD and total mortality in the first 2 years of follow-up. For the more extended 5-year follow-up the relationship between blood pressure and CVD and total mortality became positive (Taylor *et al.*, 1991) (Fig. 2.6). The results from these two large studies provide strong confirmation for the hypothesis that the association between blood pressure and mortality in later life is obscured by concurrent illness lowering blood pressure rather than a low pressure itself being a risk factor for mortality.

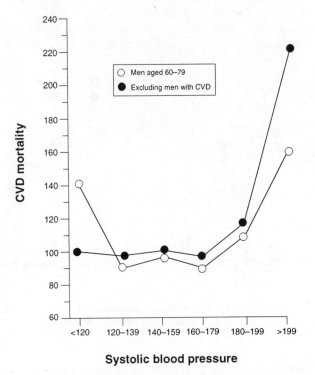

Fig. 2.5   Systolic blood pressure and cardiovascular disease (CVD) mortality

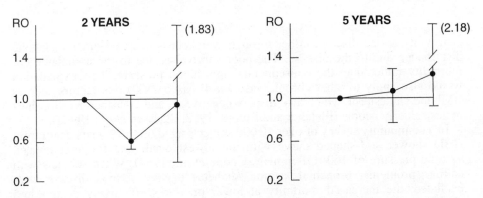

Fig. 2.6   Two- and five-year follow-up of the relationship between blood pressure and cardio-vascular disease mortality

The SHEP trial in elderly subjects with isolated systolic hypertension also provides reassurance that low diastolic pressures can be safely reduced (SHEP, 1991). In actively treated patients the reductions in systolic pressures from an average of 171 mmHg to 142 mmHg accompanied by a lowering of diastolic pressure from 77 mmHg to 68 mmHg were associated with a significant 27%

reduction in myocardial infarction. 60% of patients had baseline ECG abnormalities and in these the reduction in CHD events was 31%. The mean blood pressure of these patients with treated isolated systolic hypertension was still high and therefore these results may not necessarily be extrapolated to subjects with lower systolic and diastolic pressures.

CONCLUSIONS

In most societies, the rise in blood pressure with age leads to a substantial proportion of elderly people with blood pressures in the range usually considered for antihypertensive therapy. In the UK, approximately half the general practitioner consultations in the 65 to 74 age group are for uncomplicated hypertension, while in the over 75s, heart failure and hypertension equally account for half the consultations (RCGP, 1986). The elderly are also the highest consumers of medicines: surveys of prescription use in the elderly in the UK found that 25% of 65 to 74 year olds and nearly 40% of the over 75s were taking diuretics; comparable figures for beta-blockers and vasodilators in the over 65s were 15% and 7% (Cartwright and Smith, 1988). It is likely that antihypertensive indications account for at least half these prescriptions. Increasing evidence from randomised trials (see Chapter 4) of the benefits of treating both systolic and diastolic pressures in elderly people are likely to further increase the proportions of elderly people receiving treatment. The economic costs of treating hypertension are likely to rise even further in the future because of the increasing numbers of elderly people in the population. There is, at present, little ground for optimism in the UK that future cohorts of elderly people will have lower blood pressures even though the reduction of mean systolic blood pressure by 5 mmHg between 1991/2 to 2005 is a Health of the Nation target (DoH, 1992). Population strategies for lowering blood pressure (weight reduction, low salt and reduced alcohol intake) have not been evaluated and results from the North Karelia Salt study did not suggest grounds for optimism from salt restriction (Nissinen *et al.*, 1992). Moreover, measurements of BMI in the UK population suggest a worrying trend to higher BMIs. Hypertension in elderly people is likely to remain a major health and economic burden for the foreseeable future.

REFERENCES

Amery A, Birkenhager W, Bulpitt CJ *et al.* 1991. Syst-Eur. A multicentre trial on the treatment of isolated systolic hypertension in the elderly: Objectives, protocol and organization. *Aging Clinical and Experimental Research* **3**, 287–302.

Applegate WB, Davis BR, Black HR, McFate Smith W, Miller ST, Burlando AJ 1991. Prevalence of postural hypotension at baseline in the Systolic Hypertension in the Elderly Program (SHEP) cohort. *Journal of the American Geriatrics Society* **39**, 1057–64.

Aronow WS, Herzig AH, Fritzner E, D'Alba P, Ronquillo J 1989. 40 month follow up of risk factors correlated with new coronary events in 708 elderly patients. *Journal of the American Geriatrics Society* **37**, 501–6.

Barker DG, Osmond G, Golging J, Kuh D, Wadsworth ME 1989. Growth in utero, blood pressure in childhood and adult life and mortality from cardiovascular disease. *British Medical Journal* **298**, 564–7.

Beevers DG 1988. Overtreating hypertension. *British Medical Journal* 297, 1212–13.

Bulpitt CJ, Palmer AJ, Fletcher AE *et al.* 1992. Relation between treated blood pressure and death from ischaemic heart disease at different ages: a report from the Department of Health and Hypertension Care Computing project. *Journal of Hypertension* 10, 1273–8.

Cartwright A, Smith C 1988. *Elderly people, their medicines and their doctors.* London: Routledge.

Chiang B, Perlman L, Epstein F 1969. Overweight and hypertension: a review. *Circulation* 89, 413–21.

Colandrea MA, Friedman GD, Nichaman MZ, Lynd CN 1970. Systolic hypertension in the elderly: an epidemiologic assessment. *Circulation* 41, 239–45.

Coope J, Warrender TS 1987. Lowering blood pressure. *Lancet* ii, 518.

Coope J, Warrender TS, McPherson K 1988. The prognostic significance of blood pressure in the elderly. *Journal of Human Hypertension* 2, 79–88.

Cruickshank JM, Thorpe JM, Zacharias FJ 1987. Benefits and potential harm of lowering blood pressure. *Lancet* i, 581–4.

Department of Health 1992. *Specification of national indicators.* London: HMSO.

Dyer AR, Elliott P 1989. The INTERSALT study: relations of body mass index to blood pressure. *Journal of Human Hypertension* 3, 299–308.

Elliott P 1991. Observational studies on salt and blood pressure. *Hypertension* 17, 13–18.

Epstein FH, Eckoff RD 1967. The epidemiology of high blood pressure: Geographic distributions and aetiological factors. In Stamler J, Stamler R, Pulman TN (eds), *The epidemiology of hypertension.* New York: Grune & Stratton, 155–66.

Fagard RH 1993. Physical fitness and blood pressure. *Journal of Hypertension* 11(Suppl. 5), S47–52.

Fletcher AE, Bulpitt CJ 1992. Epidemiological aspects of cardiovascular disease in the elderly. *Journal of Hypertension* 10(Suppl. 2), S51–8.

Fortmann SP, Haskell WL, Vranizan K, Brown BW, Farquhar JW 1983. The association of blood pressure and dietary alcohol: differences by age, sex and oestrogen use. *American Journal of Epidemiology* 118, 497–507.

Harris T, Cook E, Kannel WB, Goldman L 1988. Proportional hazards analysis of risk factors for coronary heart disease in individuals aged 65 or older. *Journal of the American Geriatrics Society* 36, 1023–8.

Kannel WB, Gordon T 1978. Evaluation of cardiovascular risk in the elderly: The Framingham Study. *Bulletin of the New York Academy of Medicine* 54, 573–91.

Klatsky AL, Friedman GD, Spieglaub AB, Gerard MJ 1977. Alcohol consumption and blood pressure. Kaiser Permanent Multiphasic Health Examination Data. *New England Journal of Medicine* 296, 1194–2000.

Langer RD, Ganiats BG, Barret-Connor E 1989. Paradoxical survival of elderly men with high blood pressure. *British Medical Journal* 298, 1356–8.

Law CM, Barker DG 1994. Foetal influences on blood pressure. *Journal of Hypertension* 12, 1329–32.

Law MR, Frost CD, Wald NJ 1991a. By how much does dietary salt reduction lower blood pressure. I – Analysis of observational data among populations. *British Medical Journal* 312, 811–15.

Law MR, Frost CD, Wald NJ 1991b. By how much does dietary salt reduction lower blood pressure. II – Analysis of observational data within populations. *British Medical Journal* 312, 815–18.

Lindholm L, Lanke J, Bengtsson B 1986. U shaped associations between mortality and blood pressure in a 13 year prospective study. *Family Practice* 3, 3–8.

Macrae AD, Bulpitt CJ 1989. Assessment of postural hypotension in elderly patients. *Age and Ageing* 18, 110–12.

Mattila K, Haavisto M, Rajala S, Heikinheimo R 1988. Blood pressure and five year survival in the very old. *British Medical Journal* 296, 887–9.

McMahon S, Peto R, Cutler J *et al.* 1990. Blood pressure, stroke and coronary heart disease. Part 1, prolonged differences in blood pressure: prospective observational studies corrected for the regression dilution bias. *Lancet* **335**, 765–74.

Miall WE, Greenberg G 1987. *Mild hypertension – is there pressure to treat?* Cambridge: Cambridge University Press.

Miall WE, Lovell HG 1967. Relationship between change of blood pressure and age. *British Medical Journal* **2**, 660–4.

Nissinen A, Tuomilheto J, Enlund H, Kottke TE 1992. Costs and benefits of community programmes for the control of hypertension. *Journal of Human Hypertension* **6**, 473–9.

O'Brien E, Murphy J, Tyndall A *et al.* 1991. Twenty four hour ambulatory blood pressure in men and women aged 17 to 80 years: the Allied Irish Bank Study. *Journal of Hypertension* **9**, 335–60.

OPCS Social Survey Division 1994. *Health survey for England 1993*. London: HMSO.

Paffenberger RS, Wing AL, Hyde RT, Jung DL 1983. Physical activity and incidence of hypertension in college alumni. *American Journal of Epidemiology* **117**, 245–57.

Poulter NR, Khaw KT, Hopwood BEC *et al.* 1990. The Kenyan Luo migrant study: observations on the initiation of a rise in blood pressure. *British Medical Journal* **300**, 967–72.

Poulter NR, Khaw KT, Mugambi M, Peart WS, Rose G, Sever PS 1985. Blood pressure patterns in relation to age, weight and urinary electrolytes in three Kenyan communities. *Transactions of the Royal Society for Tropical Medicine and Hygiene* **79**, 389–92.

Rimm EB, Giovannucci EL, Willett WC *et al.* 1991. Prospective study of alcohol consumption and risk of coronary disease in men. *Lancet* **338**, 464–8.

Royal College of General Practitioners, Office of Population Censuses and Surveys, Department of Health and Social Security 1986. *Morbidity statistics from general practice 1981–1982, Series MB5 no. 1*. London: HMSO.

Rutan GH, Hermanson B, Bild DE, Kittner SJ, LaBaw F, Tell GS 1992. Orthostatic hypotension in older adults. The cardiovascular health study. *Hypertension* **19**, 508–19.

Shaper AG 1967. Blood pressure studies in east Africa. In Stamler J, Stamler R, Pullman TN (eds), *The epidemiology of hypertension*. New York: Grune & Stratton.

SHEP Cooperative Research Group 1991. Prevention of stroke by antihypertensive drug treatment in older persons with isolated systolic hypertension. *Journal of the American Medical Association* **265**, 3255–64.

Staessen J, Amery A, Birkenhager W *et al.* 1990a. Is a high serum cholesterol associated with longer survival in elderly hypertensives? *Journal of Hypertension* **8**, 755–61.

Staessen J, Amery A, Fagard R 1990b. Isolated systolic hypertension in the elderly. *Journal of Hypertension* **8**, 393–405.

Staessen J, Bulpitt C, Clement D *et al.* 1989. The relationship between mortality and treated blood pressure in elderly patients with hypertension: report of the European Working Party on High Blood Pressure in the Elderly. *British Medical Journal* **298**, 1552–6.

Stamler R, Stamler J, Riedlinger WF, Algera G, Roberts RH 1978. Weight and blood pressure: findings in hypertension screening of 1 million Americans. *Journal of the American Medical Association* **240**, 1607–10.

Svardsudd K, Tibblin G 1980. A longitudinal blood pressure study: change of blood pressure during 10 years in relation to initial values: the study of men born in 1913. *Journal of Chronic Disease* **33**, 627–36.

Swales JD 1995. *Special subgroups in manual of hypertension*. Chapter 7. Oxford: Blackwell Science.

Systolic Hypertension in the Elderly Program 1993. Implications of the systolic hypertension in the elderly program. *Hypertension* **21**, 335–43.

Taylor JO, Cornoni-Huntley J, Curb JD *et al.* 1991. Blood pressure and mortality risk in the elderly. *American Journal of Epidemiology* **134**, 489–501.

Veerman DP, Imholz BP, Wieling W, Karemaker JM, van Montfrans GA 1994. Effects of aging on blood pressure variability in resting conditions. *Hypertension* **24**, 120–30.

Whelton PK, He Jiang, Klag MJ 1994. Blood pressure in Westernised populations. In Swales JD (ed.), *Textbook of hypertension*. Oxford: Blackwell Scientific Publications, 11–21.

Woodhouse PR, Khaw Kay-Tee, Plummer M 1993. Seasonal variation of blood pressure and its relationship to ambient temperature in an elderly population. *Journal of Hypertension* **11**, 1267–74.

World Hypertension League 1991. Alcohol and hypertension: implications for management. *Bulletin of the World Health Organisation* **69**(**4**), 377–82.

Worynarowska B, Mukherjee D, Roche AF, Siervogel RM 1985. Blood pressure changes during adolescence and subsequent adult blood pressure level. *Hypertension* **7**, 695–701.

CHAPTER 3

Pathogenesis of hypertension

DAVID TUNBRIDGE

INTRODUCTION

If you can model the control of the circulation then you must have a good under-standing of the process (Casti, 1992). The study of hypertension has reached that position. Blood pressure is a physiological measurement, it therefore follows that the model represents physiological processes. Much of the evidence for the mechanisms underlying hypertension comes from animal work and experiments in younger patients and volunteers. Nevertheless, the principles are probably the same for older patients and specific studies in the elderly are used where possible.

Figure 3.1 identifies the key components involved in the maintenance of blood pressure. The contributions from, and interactions between, these components will be discussed.

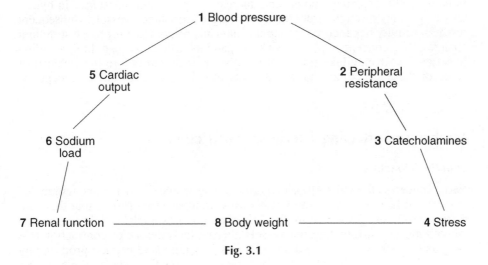

Fig. 3.1

BLOOD PRESSURE

Clinical blood pressure refers to measurements of arterial blood pressure in the upper arm using auscultatory methods. The limitations of this methodology are well known but often overlooked in practice (Petrie *et al.*, 1990).

The first step in the modelling of hypertension is to define blood pressure as the product of cardiac output and peripheral resistance. Haemodynamic studies have consistently shown that in established hypertension the abnormality is an increase in peripheral resistance (Heagerty *et al.*, 1993; Mulvany 1993). The increase in peripheral resistance remains a feature of hypertension in the elderly. In research terms this gives direction to the search for causes of hypertension, and in practice, supports the selection of antihypertensive drugs that reduce peripheral resistance (McCoy, 1993).

PERIPHERAL RESISTANCE

Within the arterial tree the vessels that make the major contribution to peripheral resistance are at arteriolar level (Mulvany, 1993). Factors which contribute to the constriction of these resistance vessels need to be incorporated into the model.

In pathological processes the time-scale of events is a crucial feature. Experimental data strictly applies only to the time period of the experiment, yet clinical hypertension is a process which develops over a period of years (Fletcher *et al.*, 1992; Gillman *et al.*, 1993; Stamler *et al.*, 1993). The difficulty of carrying out experiments over a time-scale appropriate to the pace of pathological changes hampers the study of hypertension.

Structural change in resistance vessels

Folkow (1990) explained the chronic increase in peripheral resistance in hypertensive patients through structural narrowing of resistance vessels. Subsequent research activity has focused on the mechanisms responsible for these structural changes. His concept explains why, in patients who have had long-standing hypertension, it may take up to 18 months of treatment before the reversal of some of these structural changes permits blood pressure to fall to acceptable levels.

Mechanisms affecting arteriolar constriction

Endothelial factors

Early concepts divided causes of peripheral resistance into factors within the vessels and factors outwith the vessels. Research has since shown that there are factors produced from within the endothelium of vessels which act on the smooth muscle surrounding the vessels altering their degree of contraction (De Mey and Schiffers, 1993). Endothelin-1 is a 21 amino acid peptide produced by endothelial cells, with 75% of it being released on the side of the vascular smooth muscle cells causing vasoconstriction (Levin, 1995).

Other complex systems also operate, e.g. angiotensin I is taken up from the blood and converted into angiotensin II within the vessel wall where it has trophic as well as vasoconstricting properties. Such factors are short acting; it is not experimentally possible to determine their influence over long time periods.

These intrinsic control mechanisms might play a part in the local autoregulation of blood supply but may not contribute to long-term elevation of blood pressure.

Elastic fibres

These are characteristic of medium and large arteries. Loss of elastic tissue function with increasing age results in the more distal parts of the arterial tree being subjected to greater pulse pressures as the damping effect of the arterial tree is reduced through this loss of arterial compliance. High systolic pressures are characteristic of hypertension in the elderly. The resulting high end systolic stress causes left ventricular hypertrophy and increased risk of heart attack as well as stroke (Safar and London, 1994).

Changes in vascular smooth muscle

Both the loss of large artery compliance with age (McCoy, 1993) or any cause of sustained increase in blood pressure will result in an increase in the strain imposed on the vascular smooth muscle that surrounds resistance vessels. Striated muscle subjected to an increased load undergoes hypertrophy. Smooth muscle may respond by an increase in rates of growth and proliferation (Baumbach and Ghoneim, 1993; Heagerty *et al.*, 1993).

Vasodilators

More research emphasis has been placed on the study of vasoconstrictor mechanisms than on vasodilator activity. The diameter of resistance vessels reflects the interaction between vasoconstrictor and vasodilator factors, so there is no reason why certain causes of hypertension might not be the result of a failure of vasodilator mechanisms.

Nitric oxide (NO)

Meticulous research techniques have shown that NO can be produced within cells. Although it has a half-life of only microseconds and is released continuously (Rubanyi *et al.*, 1986), it is a sufficiently powerful vasodilator to be considered a major influence on smooth muscle contraction. There is indirect evidence to suggest that the basal formation of NO is reduced in patients with hypertension (Vallance *et al.*, 1989).

Acetylcholine

The vasodilator properties of acetylcholine appear to be dependent on endothelial function (Feletou and Vanhoutte, 1988; Furchgott and Zawadzki, 1980). Anatomical studies have shown morphological changes in the endothelium in the presence of hypertension. This vasodilator action of acetylcholine has been reported as being impaired in proportion to the duration and severity of hypertension (Luscher *et al.*, 1987).

Kinins

These polypeptides are produced from the breakdown of circulating kininogen and induce vasodilation through the release of endothelial components

(Shimamoto and Iimura, 1992). Breakdown of bradykinin is partly controlled by converting enzyme (Kolber-Postepska *et al.*, 1994). Converting enzyme inhibitors that block conversion of angiotensin I to angiotensin II also inhibit the breakdown of bradykinin. The resulting rise in kinin levels might contribute to the cardioprotective action of converting enzyme inhibitors (Nolly *et al.*, 1994).

Atrial natriuretic peptide (ANP)

One hormone may often have different actions at different tissue sites. ANP elegantly links separate components of the physiological model of hypertension by exhibiting complementary forms of action on different tissues. Thus it has a vasodilator action on vascular smooth muscle and a natriuretic effect on renal tubules, both these actions serving to reduce blood pressure. However, ANP probably only operates in situations of circulatory overload (Deutsch *et al.*, 1994; Richards *et al.*, 1995).

THE AUTONOMIC NERVOUS SYSTEM – NEUROGENIC EFFECTS

The release of noradrenaline at sympathetic nerve terminals is known to be one factor through which regional circulation is modified. This occurs in response to sudden changes in cardiac output as monitored by the stretch receptors of the heart and carotid arteries.

Circulating plasma noradrenaline levels, along with systolic blood pressure, tend to increase with age. This might reflect no more than a compensatory increase in sympathetic activity in relation to the fall in cardiac output that also occurs with increasing age. This increase in sympathetic activity might, through the trophic action of catecholamines, contribute towards the structural changes in resistance vessels (Esler *et al.*, 1989).

STRESS

The activity of the sympathetic system is also influenced by higher centres within the brain. Increased noradrenaline release at sympathetic nerve terminals can be detected in experimental subjects by provocations as small as the prospect of a test of mental arithmetic. It is unclear how these short-term increases in blood pressure levels relate to the development of sustained hypertension in later life.

Because hypertension occurs during acute stress it has been postulated that chronic stress is a potential cause of chronic hypertension. Rats genetically pre-disposed to hypertension develop more severe hypertension when subjected to chronic stress but the stress effect is much less marked in normotensive strains. Once more the research methodology is not available to determine the long-term consequences of stress in human populations (Julius *et al.*, 1991).

GENETICS

Although Platt showed the strong familial pattern of hypertension, it was Pickering who won the argument that, in large populations, hypertension was normally distributed. Geneticists recognise that the pattern of inheritance in hypertension suggests a polygenic process (Bell, 1993; Dudley *et al.*, 1992; Kurtz and Spence, 1993; Schieken, 1993). They are now confident that abnormalities in the genes coding for mechanisms known to control blood pressure will be found, and that such abnormalities will explain hypertension of a familial pattern (Lifton and Jeunemaitre, 1993). As it becomes possible to identify abnormalities by genetic markers within specific control systems, it might also become possible to tailor drug therapy to counteract the defined abnormality, or at least enable us to provide a better assessment of the risks of hypertension to individuals with particular genotypes.

CARDIAC OUTPUT

Although haemodynamic studies in chronic hypertension have identified an increase in peripheral resistance rather than an increase in cardiac output as the cause of chronic hypertension, the regulation of cardiac output in relation to this sustained increase in afterload is an important factor in determining the resulting blood pressure. As blood pressure is the product of cardiac output and peripheral resistance, cardiac output is the product of heart rate and stroke volume.

Heart rate

This variable, at least, is easily measured. In young patients with hypertension it is commonly elevated. Such individuals often have 'labile hypertension', 'white-coat hypertension', an increased 'defence reaction' and on repeated measurement both their blood pressure and pulse rate 'regress towards the mean'.

This reactivity of the circulatory system has been attributed to over-activity of the sympathetic nervous system mediated through higher centres. The beta activity of adrenaline increases both the rate and force of cardiac contraction, while the alpha activity increases the peripheral resistance.

It has been postulated, but not proved, that labile hypertension in young individuals initiates circulatory changes which result in sustained hypertension and an increase in cardiovascular deaths in later life (Gillman *et al.*, 1993; Lund-Johansen, 1989).

Stroke volume

Sustained hypertension implies effective left ventricular function. The increase in deaths from heart disease in hypertensive patients does, however, focus attention on cardiac function. The increase in afterload as a result of sustained hypertension provides an increased workload on the left ventricle, which produces compensatory hypertrophy of the left ventricle. This process mirrors the duration and severity of the hypertension. Left ventricular hypertrophy is assessed by the position and force of the apex beat, electrophysiologically through ECG changes and by ultrasound measurements of left ventricular wall thickness.

Without treatment to lower the blood pressure this process would result in acute left ventricular failure. With effective hypotensive treatment acute left ventricular failure becomes unlikely and left ventricular wall thickness can revert towards normal (Nakashima *et al.*, 1984; Strauer *et al.*, 1984).

Detection of left ventricular hypertrophy, however, still conveys a poor prognosis (Grossman and Messerli, 1992). One concept is that the increased thickness of the cardiac muscle, coupled with increased oxygen requirements as a result of the increased cardiac workload, makes the cardiac muscle more susceptible to ischaemic injury (Devereux and Roman, 1993; Webster *et al.*, 1993). The role of the left ventricle in maintaining hypertension is certainly observed in hypertensive patients who suffer a myocardial infarction. The resulting impaired left ventricular function is marked by a fall in blood pressure. The time taken for blood pressure to rise first to normal levels and then again for the patient to become hypertensive is a measure of the adaptive response of the left ventricle after ischaemic damage. It can take up to 6 months before hypertension returns.

Control of stroke volume

In severe hypertension the ejection fraction falls as the left ventricle fails to empty against high aortic pressure. The primacy of increased peripheral resistance in hypertension is again seen in that despite this reduction in stroke volume in patients with severe hypertension their hypertension persists.

In this situation other compensatory mechanisms come into operation. In patients with accelerated hypertension the high blood pressure causes increased glomerular filtration and circulatory fluid is lost. Volume receptors trigger the renin–angiotensin–aldosterone system and the resulting increase in angiotensin II levels promotes hypertension while the increase in aldosterone secretion reduces renal sodium loss but increases renal potassium excretion. The extent to which these changes influence blood pressure have been shown in experiments where an infusion of saline to patients with accelerated hypertension have resulted in a reduction in blood pressure.

In sustained hypertension the effects on the heart are all due to the increase in afterload. The situation is different in patients with acute renal failure where circulatory volume commonly increases and central venous pressure is increased. An increase in pre-load will result in an increase in ANP production and a reduction in angiotensin II production but neither of these compensatory mechanisms is usually sufficient to stop blood pressure rising.

SODIUM LOAD

The renal handling of sodium excretion in patients with hypertension has been extensively studied. In general, patients with hypertension excrete an intravenous sodium load more rapidly than normotensives. This would indicate a compensatory response. Such a compensatory response can be impaired in elderly hypertensives because of the gradual loss of nephrons due to ageing.

The handling of oral sodium loads has been more difficult to study. A large reduction in sodium load does result in a small reduction in blood pressure. Populations show variations in the sensitivity of their blood pressure response to sodium loads; this again points to genetic variations in the operation of sodium regulating mechanisms (Weinberger, 1993).

The renin–angiotensin–aldosterone system affects blood pressure control through its influence on sodium balance and vasoconstrictor tone (Laragh, 1993). Pathological excess of renin produced from the exceedingly rare renin secreting tumours or of aldosterone from adrenal adenomas does result in sustained hypertension. This system can be activated in severe hypertension as previously described. In more moderate sustained hypertension the system is less active, indicating an appropriate compensatory adjustment. An argument can be made that the response, although compensatory, is not sufficient as drugs which block the action of angiotensin II and of aldosterone are effective in lowering blood pressure.

Diuretics act as powerful stimuli to the renin–angiotensin–aldosterone system but still effectively lower blood pressure in elderly patients. The fact that they would lower blood pressure more effectively without this compensatory response is shown by the marked fall in blood pressure when the compensatory angiotensin II production is blocked by the introduction of an angiotension-converting enzyme inhibitor (ACE inhibitor).

In elderly patients, as systolic blood pressures tend to rise with age, the resting levels of renin tend to fall. This again indicates a compensatory rather than causative response.

RENAL FUNCTION

Approximately 10% of patients with sustained hypertension will have some evidence of renal abnormality (McClellan, 1993; Ruilope, 1993). Microalbuminuria is commonly found in patients with hypertension (Ruilope et al., 1992). Interestingly, this proved to be a better marker for the risk of associated vascular disease than as a marker for primary renal disease (Rambausek et al., 1992). Albuminuria is a stronger marker of the presence of additional renal disease. Hypertension associated with intrinsic renal disease carries a poor prognosis as it follows the natural history of the underlying renal disease.

The influence of renal function on hypertension is through alterations in the regulation of fluid balance. Only small alterations are required to exert large influences on blood pressure. Renal function, as measured by changes in creatinine clearance, declines with age (Lakatta et al., 1993). This decline is more marked in patients who also have hypertension (Grossman and Messerli, 1992). The interdependence of blood pressure and renal function is therefore seen to an even greater extent in elderly patients.

OBESITY

There is a strong relationship between body weight and blood pressure in young patients but the effect lessens with increasing age (Julius et al., 1990). The majority of mature patients treated for hypertension are overweight. The position is not dissimilar to that found with type II diabetics (Resnick, 1992). A reduction in weight by 6 kg results on average in a 9 mmHg fall in diastolic blood pressure.

The metabolic links between obesity and hypertension are uncertain. An increased calorie intake is often accompanied by an increase in sodium intake. A high calorie intake promotes catecholamine production and insulin secretion. The picture of obesity, hypertension, insulin resistance and raised plasma cholesterol levels has been labelled as syndrome X (Brands and Hall, 1992; Edelson and Sowers, 1993). Given the lack of understanding concerning the aetiology of the separate components of this syndrome it is not surprising that it proves difficult to investigate in its entirety.

Body weight tends to increase with age in both men and women. In women the increase is more marked after pregnancy and again at the menopause. In men weight gain is more rapid in the 45 to 55 age range. With the over 85 age group average weights fall. This may be no more than the 'life table' effect from which it would be expected that individuals with lower than average body weight have longer than average life expectancy.

BAROCEPTOR CONTROL (REFLEX CONTROL)

Autoregulation of the circulation operates at a series of different levels. The micro-circulation in capillary beds is not a factor involved in the control of systemic blood pressure but it does provide a model, in miniature, of the auto-regulation of blood flow which involves a changing balance between local metabolic demands, temperature control, and the quality and quantity of blood flow to that part of the circulation. This is one effect contributing to the degree of coronary reserve (Devereux and Roman, 1993; Motz *et al.*, 1993).

Part of the regulation in regional blood flow is through the activity of the sympathetic nervous system. This involves afferent and central components which influence the release of noradrenaline at sympathetic nerve terminals.

A major component in the neurogenic control of blood pressure is that of the carotid body. Sensors within the carotid body respond to changes in pulse pressure. The afferent arm of the sympathetic system conveys the response of the pressure receptors to the brain stem. This control centre then regulates both sympathetic and cholinergic activity within the autonomic system to regulate blood pressure. A simple re-setting of baroceptor sensitivity could therefore explain sustained changes in blood pressure levels. Study of the response of this system, however, indicates that it operates in the short-term control of fluctuations in blood pressure, but that in the presence of sustained changes in blood pressure, signalling from the baroceptors reverts to baseline levels of activity. Experimental removal of the carotid body results in a short-lived surge in blood pressure before it settles to normal limits.

The baroceptor mechanism is one defence against postural hypotension. Falls as a result of postural hypotension make elderly patients vulnerable to accidents. The use of alpha-blocking drugs that predispose to postural hypotension should therefore be used cautiously, if at all, in the elderly hypertensive patient.

Although the obvious mechanism of hypertension is raised peripheral resistance, the primary underlying cause is uncertain. Renal factors, central autonomic mechanisms and other effects as previously discussed play a part. Clearly, further research is required both in terms of the underlying cause and how this leads to clinical complications.

COMPLICATIONS OF HYPERTENSION

Introduction

The complications of hypertension result from arterial damage and cardiac hypertrophy. These changes are a product of the severity and duration of the hypertension (Anversa *et al.*, 1992).

However, once blood pressure reaches 'malignant levels' the rate of damage is accelerated. Such damage is evident in the arteries within the retina and the renal glomerulae and can result in permanent loss of vision and deteriorating renal function (Rambausek *et al.*, 1992). Successful detection and treatment of hypertension in the UK has resulted in a marked reduction in the incidence of malignant hypertension (Pampalon, 1993).

Hypertension affects all sizes of arteries from branch retinal arteries to the aorta (Zanchetti *et al.*, 1993). The pathological changes resulting from hypertension affect all layers of the artery from the endothelium to the adventitia.

Atheroma

The endothelial changes can be summarised as an increased prevalence of atheromatous plaques. The associated reduction of the arterial lumen in medium sized vessels results in an increased risk of cardiac and cerebral thrombosis. Atheromatous plaques in hypertensive patients are at risk of rupturing, causing local dissection of the vessel wall and the risk of arterial haemorrhage.

Atheroma and hypertension are therefore overlapping conditions to the extent that elderly patients with hypertension are all likely to have extensive atheromatous changes in their arterial tree. This is made evident by the excess in deaths from ischaemic heart disease as well as stroke in hypertensive patients and the high incidence of peripheral vascular disease.

The major factors apart from hypertension that promote the development of atheroma are well known and outside the scope of this chapter (Ostrow and Miller, 1993). Because of the overlap between hypertension and atheroma, consideration of a family history of ischaemic heart disease, smoking habits (Payne *et al.*, 1993) and prevailing cholesterol level (Hames *et al.*, 1993; Kaiser, 1993) should be considered when managing hypertension in order to reduce the risks from these associated complications (Kannel, 1993).

Cardiac complications

Hypertension affects the heart by two mechanisms. The increase in left ventricular workload caused by hypertension initiates changes that result in left ventricular hypertrophy and its complications. The second effect is through hypertension, which promotes the development of atheroma in coronary arteries. The combination of these factors results in a high level of cardiac morbidity and mortality – almost 80% of deaths in untreated hypertensive patients.

The development of left ventricular hypertrophy is related to the severity and duration of hypertension (Anversa *et al.*, 1992). It is logical therefore that it serves as a prognostic marker in patients with hypertension (Devereux *et al.*, 1993; Dunn and Pringle, 1993; Gosse and Dallocchio, 1993; Schmieder, 1992; Zanchetti *et al.*, 1993). With the advent of effective therapy for hypertension there is evidence that these changes can be reversed (Fernandez-Alfonso *et al.*, 1992). Debate continues as to whether certain antihypertensive agents are more effective than others in reversing the changes of left ventricular hypertrophy (Clement *et al.*, 1993). Even with effective therapy the finding of left ventricular hypertrophy on echocardiographic studies still conveys an increased risk of myocardial infarction (Devereux and Roman, 1993). The progression from left ventricular hypertrophy to acute left ventricular failure as a consequence of uncontrolled hypertension is now as rare as the other potential complications of malignant hypertension. Because of improvements in the control of blood pressure, it is now unusual for patients to progress from left ventricular hypertrophy into chronic left ventricular failure, pulmonary hypertension and subsequent right ventricular failure (Schwartzkopff *et al.*, 1993).

Although improved blood pressure recognition and treatment have reduced the complications that result from impaired left ventricular function, patients with hypertension are now more likely to present with left ventricular failure and subsequent right ventricular failure as a result of myocardial damage from ischaemic heart disease. In addition to the increase in atheroma formation, it has been suggested that left ventricular hypertrophy makes the myocardium more susceptible to ischaemic damage in association with coronary artery thrombosis, and there is an increase in oxygen consumption of the left ventricle per unit of weight.

The practical reality is that more patients with hypertension now die from myocardial infarction than from all other cardiovascular causes. Patients who have experienced a transient ischaemic attack in association with carotid artery stenosis, for example, are three times more likely to die from coronary artery disease than from a stroke. The effect of treatment with thiazide diuretics and beta-blockers on the risk of cardiac disease is discussed in Chapter 4. We await the results of ongoing studies to show whether or not newer drugs such as the ACE inhibitors will be better at reducing death from myocardial infarction.

Cerebrovascular complications

Hypertension is the major risk factor for stroke. Both ischaemic and haemorrhagic stroke are associated with hypertension but haemorrhage may be more common than in the normotensive population. About 85% of strokes are atherothrombotic. A computed tomography brain scan is necessary to diagnose haemorrhage but some larger studies have classified strokes as thrombotic without the benefit of imaging. Half of stroke disease can be attributed to hypertension and effective treatment of hypertension has been shown to halve the incidence of stroke during the 3–5 year time scale of clinical trials (Besdine, 1993; Lund-Johansen, 1992; Robertson, 1992).

Again the process of atheroma is involved in the aetiology of stroke disease in hypertensive patients. One pathology associated with haemorrhagic stroke in hypertensive patients is the rupture of an atheromatous plaque as a consequence of stresses in the vessel wall caused by the pressure effects on the artery.

The prevalence of certain of these complications in relation to age was obtained by analysis of data from 450 patients attending a specialist hyper-tension clinic and is shown in Table 3.1. Cardiovascular symptoms and events show a marked increase in prevalence with increasing age. By comparison the prevalence of dyspepsia and asthma vary little across the decades.

Table 3.1   Prevalence of complications with age

| Age by decade | Prevalence as a percentage of the age group | | | |
	'4th&5th'	'6th'	'7th'	'8th&9th'
CVA or TIA	3	13	17	34
Angina	1	16	21	28
Myocardial infarction	1	3	12	6
Claudication	1	10	23	26
Dyspepsia	21	28	24	21

Stroke is more closely associated with elevated levels of systolic rather than diastolic blood pressure (Besdine, 1993; Colquhoun, 1993; Lakatta *et al.*, 1993; Robertson, 1992). Because of increasing atheromatous deposits and increasing systolic blood pressures with age, stroke is more common in elderly hyperten-sive patients. There was initial scepticism that reducing high systolic pressures in elderly patients would be as effective at preventing stroke as in younger patients (Lakatta *et al.*, 1993). Treatment trials in the elderly have, however, shown that lowering the blood pressure does result in a reduction in the incidence of stroke (Lund-Johansen, 1992; Robertson, 1992). An important factor in these trials is that although the relative reduction in the incidence of stroke in treated patients was less than that found in trials involving younger patients, the absolute rate of stroke was 10 times higher in the elderly age group (Kannel, 1993). This makes intervention to reduce the incidence of stroke a more efficient process in the elderly as fewer patients have to be treated to effect a significant reduction in the incidence of stroke.

Retinal complications

Examination of the retina provides an opportunity to study the state of small arteries. In patients with sustained hypertension the walls of the retinal vessels increase in thickness. This is most easily observed where the retinal arteries compress the retinal veins at cross-over points. The resulting indentation of the vein by the thickened artery gives rise to the physical sign of 'AV nipping'. With further thickening of the retinal artery, the light from the ophthalmoscope is reflected along the length of the vessel, a physical sign known as 'silver wiring'.

As vessels thicken they also show increased tortuousity. These physical signs relate more to the duration of hypertension than its severity and represent the development of arteriosclerosis. They are therefore common in elderly hypertensives.

A second and less common set of signs relates more directly to the severity of the hypertension. Early changes in severe hypertension include narrowing of retinal arteries and localised spasms. Later changes reflect damage to arteries sufficient to cause leakage into, and then through, the vessel wall with resulting exudates, haemorrhage and ischaemic changes. Haemorrhage more often occurs at the bifurcation of vessels and is associated with the presence of microaneurysms.

A further manifestation of vascular damage is the development of 'exudates'. 'Hard' exudates are composed of free lipid material and lipid-containing retinal macrophages. 'Cotton-wool spots' have been shown to mark areas of focal retinal ischaemia brought about by occlusion of terminal retinal arterioles (Hayreh *et al.*, 1989). Papilloedema in patients with severe hypertension was considered to be a manifestation of raised intracranial pressure. Experimental study of papilloedema has shown that the oedema can be produced as a result of relative occlusion of the arterial supply to the nerve head (Tso and Jampol, 1982). These retinal changes provided a useful prognostic guide before adequate therapy for hypertension became available.

Ophthalmic surgeons refer patients with retinal vein occlusion to physicians for evaluation of their associated hypertension (Rath *et al.*, 1992). The link between these conditions can be explained by compression of the vein by the thickened overlying artery (Keenan *et al.*, 1993). The resulting retinal ischaemia can give rise to neo-vascularisation similar to that seen in diabetic retinopathy.

In elderly hypertensive patients there is an increased incidence of high pressure glaucoma (Dielemans *et al.*, 1995).

Renal complications

Chicken or egg?

The assessment of any patient with hypertension involves considering the possibility of underlying renal disease. Even a careful past medical history plus assessment of current renal function and a search for structural abnormalities of the renal tract may fail to detect primary renal disease. Surveys of hypertensive patients, however, indicate that 4% of patients will have underlying renal or renovascular disease (Berglund *et al.*, 1976; Danielson and Dammstromm, 1981) and that renovascular disease is more common in the elderly (Hansen, 1994; Scoble *et al.*, 1989).

Renal disease does, however, tend to be progressive, and although it may not be detected on the first assessment, further monitoring of renal function will detect rates of deterioration characteristic of primary renal disease. Renovascular disease can also cause progressive loss of renal function; in one survey 12% of patients became azotaemic over 42 months (Wollenweber *et al.*, 1968). The pathological mechanisms underlying such progress have been the subject of experimental study (Textor, 1994). In patients with well-controlled hypertension and no underlying renal disease, renal function can be expected to remain stable (Livingston, 1993).

Because of improvements in the detection and treatment of hypertension the incidence of malignant hypertension has fallen. Malignant hypertension is associated with direct damage to the kidney through damage to the afferent arteries and the glomerulus. The changes that can be observed in the retinal arteries also occur in the efferent arteries. The pathological lesion in the vessels is known as hyaline change; the physiological result is a loss of glomerular function. These changes are a direct result of the high pressure. Lowering the pressure reduces the risk of further damage but too great a reduction in pressure might further reduce blood flow to the glomerulae. The aim therefore is to detect patients with severe hypertension before they reach the malignant phase. Once the malignant

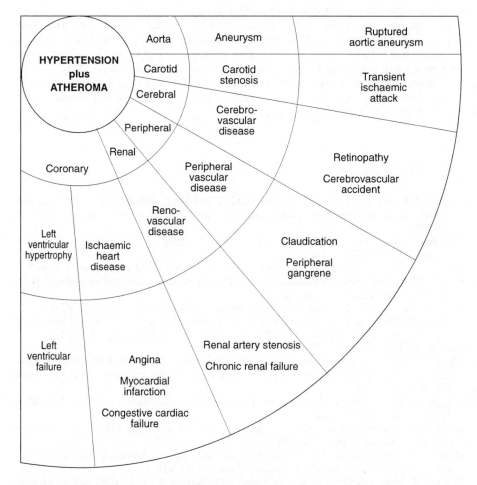

Fig. 3.2 This diagram attempts to indicate how an elderly patient with hypertension is caught in a spider's web of complications

phase is entered blood pressure has to be controlled, but a degree of irreversible renal damage may already have ensued (Webster *et al.*, 1993).

In patients with no intrinsic renal disease and in whom blood pressure is well controlled there is little chance of significant changes in renal function over time (Walker, 1993). One exception to this is when patients develop renal artery stenosis as a result of atheromatous narrowing of their renal arteries, a problem which is more common in elderly patients (Sellars *et al.*, 1985). In this situation the introduction of an ACE inhibitor or even a loop diuretic can result in a sudden fall in filtration pressure and a marked deterioration in renal function (Inman *et al.*, 1988; Speirs *et al.*, 1988). Because the primary pathology in elderly patients with renal artery stenosis is atheroma, then patients with peripheral vascular disease and femoral artery bruits are likely to have renal artery stenosis (Holley *et al.*, 1964). This association with generalised atherosclerosis is shown in that after surgical intervention for renal artery stenosis 11/15 long-term deaths were from cardiovascular causes (Van Damme *et al.*, 1995).

In conclusion, cardiac and cerebrovascular events are by far the most important complications of hypertension. Particular emphasis must be placed on developing the most effective treatment strategies to prevent these problems. Although there is now treatment to improve outcome in acute myocardial infarction, there is still no proven effective treatment for acute stroke. Prevention is clearly better than cure for these problems and hypertension is the risk factor most amenable to medical intervention.

REFERENCES

Anversa P, Capasso JM, Olivetti G, Sonnenblick EH 1992. Cellular basis of ventricular remodeling in hypertensive cardiomyopathy. *American Journal of Hypertension* **5**, 758–70.

Baumbach GL, Ghoneim S 1993. Vascular remodeling in hypertension. *Scanning Microscopy* **7**, 137–42.

Bell JI 1993. Polygenic disease. *Current Opinion in Genetics and Development* **3**, 466–9.

Berglund G, Anderson O, Wilhelmson L 1976. Prevalence of primary and secondary hypertension. *British Medical Journal* **2**, 554–6.

Besdine RW 1993. Stroke prevention in the elderly. *Connecticut Medicine* **57**, 287–92.

Brands MW, Hall JE 1992. Insulin resistance, hyperinsulinemia, and obesity-associated hypertension (editorial). *Journal of the American Society of Nephrology* **3**, 1064–77.

Casti JL 1992. *Reality rules: I.* New York: John Wiley.

Clement DL, De Buyzere M, Duprez D 1993. Left ventricular function and regression of left ventricular hypertrophy in essential hypertension. *American Journal of Hypertension* **6**(Suppl. 2), S14–19.

Colquhoun D 1993. Hypertension and heart disease. The need for clear thinking. *Australian Family Physician* **22**, 679–81.

Danielson M, Dammstromm BG 1981. The prevalence of secondary and curable hypertension. *Acta Medica Scandinavia* **209**, 451–5.

De Mey JG, Schiffers PM 1993. Effects of the endothelium on growth responses in arteries. *Journal of Cardiovascular Pharmacology* **21**(Suppl. 1), S22–5.

Deutsch A, Frishman WH, Sukenik D, Somer BG, Youssri A 1994. Atrial natriuretic peptide and its potential role in pharmacotherapy. *Journal of Clinical Pharmacology* **34**, 1133–47.

Devereux RB, de Simone G, Ganau A, Koren MJ, Roman MJ 1993. Left ventricular hypertrophy associated with hypertension and its relevance as a risk factor for complications. *Journal of Cardiovascular Pharmacology* **21**(Suppl. 2), S38–44.

Devereux RB, Roman MJ 1993. Inter-relationships between hypertension, left ventricular hypertrophy and coronary heart disease. *Journal of Hypertension* **11**(Suppl.), S3–9.

Dielemans I, Vingerling JR, Algra D, Hofman A, Grobbee DE, de Jong PT 1995. Primary open-angle glaucoma, intraocular pressure, and systemic blood pressure in the general elderly population. The Rotterdam Study. *Ophthalmology* **102**, 54–60.

Dudley CR, Giuffra LA, Reeders ST 1992. Identifying genetic determinants in human essential hypertension. *Journal of the American Society of Nephrology* **3**(Suppl. 4), S2–8.

Dunn FG, Pringle SD 1993. Sudden cardiac death, ventricular arrhythmias and hypertensive left ventricular hypertrophy. *Journal of Hypertension* **11**, 1003–10.

Edelson GW, Sowers JR 1993. Insulin resistance in hypertension: a focused review. *American Journal of Medical Science* **306**, 345–7.

Esler M, Lambert G, Jennings G 1989. The influence of ageing on catecholamine metabolism. In Amery A, Staessen J (eds), *Handbook of hypertension; hypertension in the elderly*, Vol. 12. Amsterdam: Elsevier, 85–98.

Feletou M, Vanhoutte PM 1988. Endothelium-dependent hyperpolarization of canine coronary smooth muscle. *British Journal of Pharmacology* **93**, 515–24.

Fernandez-Alfonso MS, Ganten D, Paul M 1992. Mechanisms of cardiac growth. The role of the renin-angiotensin system. *Basic Research in Cardiology* **87**(Suppl. 2), 173–81.

Fletcher AE, Bradley IC, Broxton JS *et al.* 1992. Survival of hypertensive subjects identified on screening: results for sustained and unsustained diastolic hypertension. *European Heart Journal* **13**, 1595–601.

Folkow B 1990. *Hypertension, pathophysiology, diagnosis and management.* New York: Raven Press.

Furchgott RF, Zawadzki JV 1980. The obligatory role of endothelial cells in the relaxation of arterial smooth muscle by acetylcholine. *Nature* **299**, 373–6.

Gillman MW, Kannel WB, Belanger A, D'Agostino RB 1993. Influence of heart rate on mortality among persons with hypertension: the Framingham Study. *American Heart Journal* **125**, 1148–54.

Gosse P, Dallocchio M 1993. Left ventricular hypertrophy: epidemiological prognosis and associated critical factors. *European Heart Journal* **14**(Suppl. D), 16–21.

Grossman E, Messerli FH 1992. End-organ disease in hypertension: what have we learned? *Journal of Cardiovascular Pharmacology* **20** (Suppl. 10), S1–6.

Hames CG, Rose K, Knowles M, Davis CE, Tyroler HA 1993. Black–White comparisons of 20-year coronary heart disease mortality in the Evans County Heart Study. *Cardiology* **82**, 122–36.

Hansen KJ 1994. Prevalence of ischemic nephropathy in the atherosclerotic population. *American Journal of Kidney Disease* **24**, 615–21.

Hayreh SS, Servais GE, Virdi PS 1989. Cotton wool spots (inner retinal ischemic spots) in malignant arterial hypertension. *Ophthalmologica* **198**, 197–215.

Heagerty AM, Aalkjaer C, Bund SJ, Korsgaard N, Mulvany MJ 1993. Small artery structure in hypertension. Dual processes of remodeling and growth. *Hypertension* **21**, 391–7.

Holley KE, Hunt JC, Brown AL, Kincaid OW, Sheps SG 1964. Renal artery stenosis. *American Journal of Medicine* **37**, 14–18.

Inman WHW, Rawson NSB, Wilton LV, Pearce GL, Speirs CJ 1988. Post marketing surveillance of enalapril I: results of prescription event monitoring. *British Medical Journal* **297**, 826–9.

Julius S, Jamerson K, Mejia A, Krause L, Schork N, Jones K 1990. The association of borderline hypertension with target organ changes and higher coronary risk: Tecumseh Blood Pressure Study. *Journal of the American Medical Association* **264**, 354–8.

Julius S, Jones K, Schork N *et al.* 1991. Independence of pressure reactivity from pressure levels in Tecumseh, Michigan. *Hypertension* **17**(Suppl. III), III12–21.

Kaiser FE 1993. Cholesterol and the older adult. *Southern Medical Journal* **86**(Suppl. 2), S11–14.

Kannel WB 1993. Hypertension as a risk factor for cardiac events, epidemiologic results of long-term studies. *Journal of Cardiovascular Pharmacology* **21**(Suppl. 2), S27–37.

Keenan JM, Kritzinger EE, Dodson PM 1993. Management of retinal vein occlusion. *British Journal of Hospital Medicine* **49**, 268–73.

Kolber-Postepska B, Zebrowska-Lupina I, Markiewicz M, HorubaLa-Bielak G 1994. Changes of components in the kinin system and plasma renin activity during different stages of hypertension in patients treated with captopril. *Polski Tygodnik Lekarski* **49**, 245–8.

Kurtz TW, Spence MA 1993. Genetics of essential hypertension. *American Journal of Medicine* **94**, 77–84.

Lakatta EG, Cohen JD, Fleg JL, Frohlich ED, Gradman AH 1993. Hypertension in the elderly: age and disease related complications and therapeutic implications. *Cardiovascular Drugs and Therapeutics* **7**, 643–53.

Laragh JH 1993. The renin system and new understanding of the complications of hypertension and their treatment. *Arzneimittelforschung* **43**, 247–54.

Levin ER 1995. Mechanisms of disease: Endothelins. *New England Journal of Medicine* **333**, 356–63.

Lifton RP, Jeunemaitre X 1993. Finding genes that cause human hypertension. *Journal of Hypertension* **11**, 231–6.

Livingston IL 1993. Renal disease and Black Americans: selected issues. *Social Science and Medicine* **37**, 613–21.

Lund-Johansen P 1989. Central haemodynamics in essential hypertension at rest and during exercise: a 20-year follow up study. *Journal of Hypertension* **7**(Suppl. 6), S52–5.

Lund-Johansen P 1992. Treatment of hypertension in the elderly – what have we learned from the recent trials? *Cardiovascular Drugs and Therapeutics* **6**, 571–3.

Luscher TF, Vanhoutte PM, Raij L 1987. Antihypertensive treatment normalizes decreased endothelium-dependent relaxations in rats with salt-induced hypertension. *Hypertension* **9**, III 193–7.

McClellan W 1993. Hypertensive end-stage renal disease in blacks: the role of end-stage renal disease surveillance. *American Journal of Kidney Disease* **21**(Suppl. 1), 25–30.

McCoy CE 1993. Hypertension in the elderly. *Rhode Island Medical Journal* **76**, 239–42.

Motz W, Vogt M, Strauer BE 1993. Coronary microcirculation in hypertensive heart disease: functional significance and therapeutic implications. *Clinical Investigation* **71**(Suppl.), S42–5.

Mulvany MJ 1993. Vascular remodelling in hypertension. *European Heart Journal* **14**(Suppl. C), 2–4.

Nakashima Y, Fouad FM, Tarazi RC 1984. Regression of left ventricular hypertrophy from systemic hypertension by enalapril. *American Journal of Cardiology* **53**, 1044–9.

Nolly H, Damiani MT, Miatello R 1994. Vascular-derived kinins and local control of vascular tone. *Brazilian Journal of Medicine and Biological Research* **27**, 1995–2011.

Ostrow PT, Miller LL 1993. Pathology of small artery disease. *Advances in Neurology* **62**, 93–123.

Pampalon R 1993. Avoidable mortality in Quebec and its regions. *Social Science and Medicine* **37**, 823–31.

Payne JN, Milner PC, Saul C, Bowns IR, Hannay DR, Ramsay LE 1993. Local confidential inquiry into avoidable factors in deaths from stroke and hypertensive disease. *British Medical Journal* **307**, 1027–30.

Petrie JC, O'Brien ET, Littler WA, de Sweit M, Dillon MJ, Padfield PI (eds) 1990. *Recommendations on blood pressure measurement*, 2nd edn. London: British Medical Journal Publications.

Rambausek M, Fliser D, Ritz E 1992. Albuminuria of hypertensive patients. *Clinical Nephrology* **38**(Suppl. 1), S40–5.

Rath EZ, Frank RN, Shin DH, Kim C 1992. Risk factors for retinal vein occlusions. A case-control study. *Ophthalmology* **99**, 509–14.

Resnick LM 1992. Cellular ions in hypertension, insulin resistance, obesity, and diabetes: a unifying theme. *Journal of the American Society of Nephrology* **3**(Suppl. 4), S78–85.

Richards AM, Nicholls MG, Espiner EA 1995. Natriuretic peptides. *Clinical Science (Colch)* **88**, 18–21.

Robertson JI 1992. The case for antihypertensive drug treatment in subjects over the age of 60. *Cardiovascular Drugs and Therapeutics* **6**, 579–83.

Rubanyi GM, Romero JC, Vanhoutte PM 1986. Flow-induced release of endothelium-derived relaxing factor. *American Journal of Physiology* **250**, H1145–9.

Ruilope LM 1993. Kidney and aetiology, pathology and management of essential hypertension. *Journal of Human Hypertension* **7**(Suppl. 1), S37–41.

Ruilope LM, Alcazar JM, Rodicio JL 1992. Renal consequences of arterial hypertension. *Journal of Hypertension* **10**(Suppl.), S85–90.

Safar ME, London GM 1994. The arterial system in human hypertension. In Swales JD (ed.), *Textbook of hypertension*, 1st edn. Oxford: Blackwell, 85–102.

Schieken RM 1993. Genetic factors that predispose the child to develop hypertension. *Pediatric Clinics of North America* **40**, 1–11.

Schmieder RE 1992. Hypertensive heart disease – significance of left ventricular hypertrophy. *Journal of Cardiovascular Pharmacology* **20**(Suppl. 6), S50–5.

Schwartzkopff B, Motz W, Vogt M, Strauer BE 1993. Heart failure on the basis of hypertension. *Circulation* **87**(Suppl.), IV66–72.

Scoble JE, Maher ER, Hamilton G, Dick R, Sweny P, Moorhead JF 1989. Atherosclerotic renovascular disease causing renal impairment – a case for treatment. *Clinics in Nephrology* **31**, 119–22.

Sellars L, Siamopoulos K, Hacking PM, Proud G, Taylor RMR, Essenhigh R 1985. Renovascular hypertension: ten years experience in a regional centre. *Quarterly Journal of Medicine* **219**, 403–16.

Shimamoto K, Iimura O 1992. The renal kallikrein-kinin system at the prehypertensive stage of hypertension. *Agents Actions* **38** (Suppl.), 287–93.

Speirs CJ, Dollery CT, Inman WHW 1988. Post marketing surveillance of enalapril II: investigation of the potential role of enalapril in deaths with renal failure. *British Medical Journal* **297**, 830–2.

Stamler J, Stamler R, Neaton JD 1993. Blood pressure, systolic and diastolic, and cardiovascular risks. US population data. *Archives of Internal Medicine* **153**, 598–615.

Strauer BE, Mahmoud MA, Bayer F, Bohn J, Motz W 1984. Reversal of left ventricular hypertrophy and improvement of cardiac function in man by nifedipine. *European Heart Journal* **5**(Suppl. F), 53–60.

Textor SC 1994. Pathophysiology of renal failure in renovascular disease. *American Journal of Kidney Disease* **24**, 642–51.

Tso MOM, Jampol LM 1982. Pathophysiology of hypertensive retinopathy. *Ophthalmology* **89**, 1132–45.

Vallance P, Collier J, Moncada S 1989. Effects of endothelium-derived nitric oxide on peripheral arteriolar tone in man. *Lancet* **2**, 997–1000.

Van Damme H, Lombet P, Creemers E, Jeusette F, Albert A, Limet R 1995. Surgery for occlusive renal artery disease: immediate and long-term results. *Acta Chirurgica Belgica* **95**, 1–10.

Walker WG 1993. Hypertension-related renal injury: a major contributor to end-stage renal disease. *American Journal of Kidney Disease* **22**, 164–73.

Webster J, Petrie JC, Jeffers TA, Lovell HG 1993. Accelerated hypertension – patterns of mortality and clinical factors affecting outcome in treated patients. *Quarterly Journal of Medicine* **86**, 485–93.

Weinberger MH 1993. Racial differences in renal sodium excretion: relationship to hypertension. *American Journal of Kidney Disease* **21**(Suppl. 1), 41–5.
Wollenweber J, Sheps S, Davis G 1968. Clinical course of atherosclerotic renovascular disease. *American Journal of Cardiology* **21**, 60–71.
Zanchetti A, Sleight P, Birkenhager WH 1993. Evaluation of organ damage in hypertension. *Journal of Hypertension* **11**, 875–82.

CHAPTER 4

Benefits of treatment

ANDREW K SCOTT

INTRODUCTION

Rational drug treatment involves choosing a drug that has proven benefit for a particular condition and an acceptable side effect profile. If we have a choice of similar treatments in terms of effectiveness then the most cost-effective should be used. Some clinicians have attempted to practise in this way for many years. Recently governments have been taking a greater interest in treatment costs and are looking for hard evidence of benefit. In the United Kingdom, advice from the Department of Health encourages purchasers of health care to concentrate on supporting only those treatments that have been proven to be effective. As providers of health care we continue to have responsibility for using the treatment we believe to be best for the individual patient, but, in addition, we have to be able to defend the use of that treatment to the purchasers of that care.

Rational drug treatment for hypertension requires consideration of the possible measures of outcome. The objective of treating hypertension, clearly, is to prevent the complications of raised blood pressure and not simply to lower blood pressure for its own sake. This raises major problems because large multicentre trials are necessary to prove that the treatment is preventing even the commonest consequences of hypertension – ischaemic heart disease and stroke. These large trials are difficult to carry out, very expensive and take a long time. This inevitably means that benefit from drug treatment can only be established after many years of use. Elderly hypertensive patients are at an advantage in this respect since the higher, untreated complication rate means that smaller numbers of patients are necessary to show benefit from treatment than in younger adults, and the trials can be conducted over a shorter period.

It is relatively easy to use proof of ability to lower blood pressure as the end point and assume that lowering blood pressure equates with a reduction in complications. However, it is evident from existing trial results that drugs with equal effect on blood pressure do not have the same effect on disease prevention. Some studies have used intermediate endpoints, such as left ventricular hypertrophy, as evidence of benefit from treatment when comparing different groups of antihypertensive agents, but this also does not equate exactly with benefit in terms of prevention of complications.

This chapter aims first to discuss the main outcome studies for the older drugs used in hypertension treatment in elderly patients. Second, the more limited published evidence for newer drugs will be considered to provide a basis for the rational choice of such drugs until more definitive evidence becomes available.

MAJOR OUTCOME STUDIES

Traditionally, old age starts on retirement at the age of 65 years. This figure is, of course, an arbitrary one and chronological age often bears little resemblance to biological age. In demographic terms, we are faced with an increase in the numbers of elderly people, especially the over 85 age group. In practical terms, physicians with an interest in elderly patients tend to see mainly patients over the age of 70 with a median age of over 80 years. For the purpose of this chapter the age of 60 has been selected on pragmatic grounds, since some of the studies of hypertension in elderly patients have recruited patients from that age.

At least 11 prospective, randomised trials which include older patients with hypertension have been published since 1972, though four of these also included younger patients. The six more recent studies will be considered in detail followed by a review of a meta-analysis of eight of the studies.

The Australian therapeutic trial in mild hypertension

This trial was performed in only four centres in Melbourne, Perth and Sydney commencing in 1973 (Australian Therapeutic Trial Management Committee, 1980, 1981). The subjects were mainly White Australian born volunteers who attended screening centres. Blood pressure (mean of two readings) was measured using random-zero or London School of Hygiene sphygmomanometers after 5 minutes rest with subjects seated. Entry to the trial was on the basis of two screening visits plus a third visit to a study-centre clinic giving a diastolic blood pressure of 95–109 mmHg with a systolic of less than 200 mmHg. Subjects were excluded if there was clinical evidence of cardiovascular disease, asthma, diabetes, gout, any potentially fatal disease or drug treatment with oral contraceptives or tricyclic antidepressants.

Suitable patients (age 30–69) were stratified by age and sex and randomly allocated to pharmacologically active treatment or placebo. Active treatment was chlorothiazide 500 mg once daily with an increase to 500 mg twice daily if necessary. This large dose of thiazide was typical of the time of the study but much higher than would be used now. Second-line treatment was with methyldopa, propranolol or pindolol. Third-line treatment was hydralazine or clonidine. The initial goal was to achieve a diastolic blood pressure of 90 mmHg but this was later reduced to 80 mmHg.

Endpoints were death from any cause subdivided into fatal cardiovascular events and other causes of death. The main non-fatal endpoints were cerebrovascular disease (thrombotic or haemorrhagic), myocardial infarction, other ischaemic heart disease and congestive cardiac failure. A trial endpoint committee was blinded as to the treatment used. The aim was to demonstrate a 30% reduction in mortality and morbidity over 5 years. This gave an estimate of 2428 subjects required but to allow for imprecision in the estimate a target of 3640 patients was agreed. Data was analysed by an on treatment approach and an intention to treat approach.

In practice, 3427 subjects were evaluated. This resulted from 104 171 subjects screened to give 3931 randomised patients, but 504 patients were excluded because blood pressure fell below the target before treatment was started. The study was terminated in 1979 and results from the whole group were published in 1980 with the results from the 582 'elderly' patients (age 60–69) published in 1981. Just over 2% of patients were lost to follow-up.

In the older group, a 39% ($P < 0.025$) reduction in trial endpoints was observed in the 293 actively treated subjects. The active and placebo groups were well matched except for systolic blood pressure and blood cholesterol levels, which were lower in the placebo group. This would be expected to reduce the relative effect of treatment. Approximately one third of patients in both groups failed to continue their allocated treatment. Side effects were rarely given as the reason for stopping treatment. Results were analysed by both 'intention to treat' and 'on treatment'. Numbers were too small to show a statistically significant difference in individual disease endpoints but there was a trend to a reduction in both cerebrovascular and ischaemic heart disease events.

Mortality and morbidity results from the European Working Party on high blood pressure in the elderly trial (EWPHE)

Although the earlier trials had shown some benefit for the treatment of hypertension in older patients there was still considerable debate as to whether it was worth treating hypertension in the elderly, particularly in less severe hypertension and if there was no evidence of end-organ damage. The EWPHE study (Amery *et al.*, 1985) results increased interest in treating older hypertensive patients in a more positive way.

The EWPHE trial was a double-blind, randomised placebo-controlled trial of antihypertensive treatment in patients over the age of 60. The study began in 1972 and involved 18 major centres in 11 European countries (counting Scotland as separate from England!). The methodology had been published in detail separately (EWPHE, 1985). Information available at the time indicated that a positive result would be more likely for cerebrovascular than for total cardiovascular events. The aim was therefore to be able to detect a 40% reduction in cerebrovascular mortality and morbidity at the 5% level of significance and to exclude that level of reduction with 90% power. Initial calculations suggested the need to recruit 600 men or 1400 women with 5 year follow-up. It later became clear that almost 70% of patients recruited were female and the numbers were recalculated to show that 850 patients followed for 8 years would achieve the desired power.

Blood pressure was measured in the arm with the highest systolic reading at the initial visit. Calibrated mercury column sphygmomanometers were used throughout the study. Three readings were made in recumbent (10 min), sitting (3 min) and standing (3 min) positions with the last measurement in each position being recorded. Elderly patients were admitted to the randomised study if they fulfilled the inclusion criteria of age over 60 and sitting blood pressure of 90–119 mmHg diastolic and 160–239 mmHg systolic. The main exclusion criteria were curable cause of hypertension, certain complications of hyper-tension (e.g. congestive heart failure, cerebral haemorrhage) and concurrent disease such as hepatitis, cirrhosis, gout, malignancy and insulin requiring diabetes.

Treatment was started with one diuretic capsule (25 mg hydrochlorothiazide plus 50 mg triamterene) daily. This was doubled if necessary after at least 2 weeks. If blood pressure was uncontrolled after at least 1 month, methyldopa was used in a dose of 250 mg daily increasing to 2 g daily if necessary.

The main specific study terminating events were death, non-fatal cerebral haemorrhage, congestive heart failure, severe increase in left ventricular hyper-trophy and blood pressure exceeding defined limits. The Steering Committee found that some preset trial endpoints had been reached by the summer of 1984. By this time, 840 evaluable patients had been randomised. Patients thus con-tinued in the double-blind trial until July 1984 or a terminating event occurred. Those survivors leaving the double-blind trial before 1984 continued to be followed-up but only date and cause of death were recorded. Just over 15% of patients were lost to follow-up but all-cause and cause-specific mortality is known in 97% of the patients.

Data were sent to the co-ordinating office every 3 months. Cause of death and other events were classified into previously defined categories, independently by two observers blinded as to the patient's treatment group. A per protocol analysis and an overall intention to treat analysis (confined to mortality) were performed.

Although this study included patients over the age of 60 without an upper age limit (the oldest was 97) the patients were concentrated in the lower half of the range with a mean age of 72 years. Around 70% of the patients were female and 35% had cardiovascular complications on admission to the trial. The mean blood pressure at entry was 182/101 in the placebo group and 183/101 in the active treatment group. By year 1 this had fallen to 172/95 and 151/88 respectively ($P < 0.001$). At 5 years these differences had been maintained – 171/95 and 150/85, respectively. The comparative percentage reduction in event rates is shown in Table 4.1. In the intention to treat analysis of death rates there was a significant reduction of 27% (95% confidence interval (CI) –46 to –1) in all cardiovascular deaths and 38% (95% CI –61 to –1) in cardiac deaths. In the per protocol analysis of terminating fatal events on randomised treatment there were 70 deaths/1000 patient years in the placebo group and 52/1000 patient years in the active treatment group, but this was not statistically significant (95% CI –45 to +1, $P = 0.077$). There were significant falls of 38% (95% CI –58 to –8) in total cardiovascular deaths, 47% (95% CI –71 to –3) in cardiac deaths and 60% (95% CI –84 to –4) in myocardial infarction deaths.

Total non-fatal cardiovascular terminating events were 20/1000 patient years in the placebo group and 8/1000 patient years in the active treatment group. This 60% reduction (95% CI –88 to –19) was highly significant ($P = 0.0064$). The benefit was mainly due to a 63% (95% CI –85 to –10) reduction in severe con-gestive cardiac failure. Fatal and non-fatal terminating events combined showed a 54% reduction for cardiac ($P = 0.0016$) and 46% reduction for cerebrovascular ($P = 0.058$) in the active treatment group.

For non-terminating events, there was a significant 52% (95% CI –76 to –7) reduction in total cerebrovascular episodes. A total of 306 patients (149 active treatment) stopped randomised treatment early. This was mainly due to being

Table 4.1 Summary of outcome results in six studies of hypertension in the elderly

	AUSTRAL	C&W	EWPHE	STOP	MRC	SHEP
Non-fatal:						
Stroke	37	27	35	38*	30	37*
MI	+18	+11	–	16	–	33*
All cardiac	10	26	9	–	13	40*
All CVS	26	26	36*	–	25*	36*
Fatal:						
Stroke	1	70*	32	73*	12	29
Cardiac	75	+1	38*	25	22	20
All CVS	61	22	27*	–	9	20
All non-CVS	+13	–	+21	–	+5	+5
All deaths	23	3	9	43*	3	13
All events:						
Stroke	34	42*	36*	47*	25*	36*
Cardiac	19	15	20	13	19	27*
All CVS	24	23*	34*	40*	17*	32*

MI, myocardial infarction; CVS, cardiovascular system.
% reduction in event rates; *P < 0.05.
References: AUSTRAL (Australian Therapeutic Trial Management Committee, 1981); C&W (Coope and Warrender, 1986); EWPHE (Amery *et al.*, 1985); STOP (Dahlof *et al.*, 1991); MRC (MRC Working Party, 1992); SHEP (SHEP Cooperative Research Group, 1991).

lost to follow-up (128; 59 active), stopping of trial medication (52; 30 active) and non-fatal intercurrent disease (38; 13 active).

The EWPHE trial was of long duration at 12 years (note that the Australian study took only 6 years despite having four times as many patients). Only 35% of the 840 patients were still in the double-blind part when it was stopped – 19% had died, 4% had a trial terminating morbid event, 5% had a terminating non-morbid event, and 36% left for other reasons. The 36% reduction in cardiovascular events is similar to that seen in the over 60s group in the Veterans Administration study (Veterans Administration Cooperative Study, 1972) and the Australian study. There also seemed to be a reduction in the case fatality rate in patients with myocardial infarction – reduced cardiac mortality with possibly increased non-fatal myocardial infarction in the treated group. This is in keeping with the Framingham study (Kannel and Dawber, 1974) but no significant change was observed in the Australian study. The reduction in severe but not mild congestive cardiac failure is suggested to be due to a lowering of left ventricular workload rather than a reduction in myocardial disease. A significant reduction in non-terminating cerebrovascular events was observed but the apparent reduction in cerebrovascular mortality did not reach statistical significance. This effect on stroke is therefore less clear than was expected from previous studies.

Unlike the Australian study the patients in this trial were recruited from clinics rather than by population screening. The patients are thus typical of those seen in routine practice. However, care would need to be taken before extrapolating the results to the whole population if screening measures become more widespread, as in the United Kingdom guidelines to general practitioners to measure blood pressure in all patients over the age of 75. Adverse effects were not a major problem though the results have been published separately from this main outcome paper (Amery *et al.*, 1978, 1982). As expected there were problems with decreased glucose tolerance and an increase in serum uric acid in patients on diuretics. Serum creatinine also increased on diuretics. Although creatinine is known to increase due to diuretics, this might have been offset by a protective effect against renal impairment due to higher blood pressure in the placebo group. Overall the authors favour active treatment for patients similar to those in this trial since benefits clearly outweighed the risk of adverse effects.

Randomised trial of treatment of hypertension in elderly patients in primary care

Hypertension is a common disease and as such will inevitably be treated mainly by general practitioners. This study was carried out entirely in primary care and should thus reflect the true situation, at least within the United Kingdom (Coope, 1982; Coope and Warrender, 1986). The authors used the availability of National Health Service fixed patient lists to recruit patients from a known population base of 13 general practices in England and Wales. This multicentre study was designed in 1975 with a pilot phase completed in 1977. Most of the centres were recruited between 1978 and 1981.

Patients aged 60–79 years attended screening clinics run by trial nurses. Seated blood pressure was measured in the left arm, after a short rest, using Hawksley random zero sphygmomanometers. Patients were randomised to active treatment or no treatment after three blood pressure readings of diastolic 105 mmHg or above or systolic 170 mmHg or above. The observation, controlled study design was chosen without placebos because it was considered that a double-blind design would have presented too many problems in this community based elderly population (e.g. long period of study, intercurrent illnesses, multiple medication, primary care doctor's close relationship with the patient and possible conflict with patient needs). Exclusion factors were: atrial fibrillation, atrio-ventricular heart block, ventricular failure, asthma, diabetes mellitus, any serious concomitant disease or blood pressure persistently above 280 mmHg systolic or 120 mmHg diastolic.

A three-step treatment protocol was used. First, use atenolol 100 mg once daily. Second, if blood pressure was greater than 170/105, add bendrofluazide 5 mg. If unable to tolerate atenolol 100 mg, try atenolol 50 mg then bendrofluazide alone. Third, if necessary add methyldopa 500 mg as a single evening dose. Patients who could not be controlled by a combination of these three drugs or who developed unacceptable side effects could be treated with any recognised drug. In the last 2 years of the trial several patients received nifedipine.

The main aim of the study was to determine whether treatment of hypertension in this age group reduced the incidence of stroke or coronary disease or affected cardiovascular or overall mortality. Secondary aims were to assess the risk of adverse drug effects and unwanted morbidity and to follow-up patients who had normal blood pressure on screening and to compare their morbidity and mortality with that of the hypertensive patients. Medical records were reviewed continuously by the trial nurses and every 6 months by two investigators from the administrative centre. A committee that was blinded as to the treatment given, decided on the status of morbid events.

The incidence of strokes and coronary events in the pilot stage of the trial suggested that a target of 4000 patient-years of observation would be necessary between the treatment and control groups. This assumed a one third reduction in either event from an estimated incidence of 15% over a 5-year period. Such a reduction has been assumed in the power calculations for most of the major studies. Analysis of the results was on an intention to treat basis. Recordable events were myocardial infarction, major stroke, minor stroke, transient ischaemic attack (TIA), congestive heart failure, atrial fibrillation, clinical gout, diabetes, non-fatal cancer, vertigo, dizzy spells and death. The major recordable events (myocardial infarction, stroke, death) were referred to the administrative centre on special forms. A questionnaire was used to assess side effects. All data were transferred annually to a central computer. Patients who reached the age of 80 and had been in the study for 5 years were excluded from further analysis. Those who left the participating practices were included until the time of departure. If a patient suffered more than one event of the same type they were counted as having only one episode. Also a fatal event cancelled out a non-fatal one of the same type. For stroke, the most serious event was counted (major > minor > TIA).

The trial was terminated in August 1985, giving a length of 7 years, comparable to the Australian study. A total of 10 718 patients (5987 women) had been screened, which was 78% of the total in the age range 60–79 on the practice lists. Exclusions were 1871 because of medical conditions and 1165 because they were already on treatment for hypertension. In addition 302 had untreated hypertension but were unwilling to take part. A total of 884 patients were recruited (419 treated; 465 control) and mean follow-up was 4.4 years. Patient-years of follow-up were close to target at 3900 (1845 treated; 2055 control). Interestingly these figures confirm the 'rule of halves', i.e. around half of the hypertensive patients in the 13 practices were not known to have hypertension (1186 unknown; 1165 known). The proportion of patients with hypertension was 22% assuming the 22% not screened did not differ significantly from those attending for screening.

As in previous studies the proportion of women was close to 70% and mean age was almost 69 years, with relatively less patients in the 75–79 group than in other 5 year bands. There were slightly more smokers (28 vs 21%) in the treated group and more left ventricular hypertrophy (ECG criteria) in the control group (8 vs 11%) but neither of these differences was statistically significant. In the treatment group, 70% were on atenolol and 60% on bendrofluazide; 7% were on bendrofluazide only and 5% on no drugs throughout most of the study. In the control group, 2% were on treatment because of a blood pressure above 280/120 and 7% were on diuretics for cardiac failure. Mean blood pressure on entry was 197/100 in the treatment group and 196/98 in the control group. During follow-up, the treated group fell to 162/78 compared with a fall to 180/89 in the controls. This difference of 18/11 between the two groups was maintained throughout the study after the first year. Goal blood pressure of less than 170 mmHg systolic was achieved in only 36% of the treated group (20%

controls) at the end of the first year but had increased to 62% (31% controls) by the eighth year. This is in keeping with observed practice when it is more difficult to achieve control of systolic than diastolic pressure in elderly patients.

The morbidity and mortality results were expressed as rate ratios for rate in treatment group/rate in control group. The only results to achieve statistical significance were a reduction in fatal stroke (rate ratio 0.3; 95% CI 0.11–0.84) and all strokes (rate ratio 0.58; 95% CI 0.35–0.96). The rate ratios for various coronary events were all close to one suggesting no effect on ischaemic heart disease.

Analysis of subsets by age at first admission to the study showed a similar reduction in total stroke for 60–69 years compared to 70–79 years though the numbers were too small to be able to show a significant difference of this magnitude. The rates for total mortality, stroke, coronary artery disease and all cardiovascular disease in the 1165 patients excluded because they were already on treatment were similar to those of the patients in the treatment arm of the trial.

The 42% reduction in all strokes is similar to other trials though the lack of significant effect on cardiac events is disappointing. Other studies have also shown a clearer benefit for stroke compared with cardiac events but the potential cardiac benefit is least in this trial. There appear to be two main differences from other studies. First, patients with low diastolic pressures were included whereas other studies (except SHEP to be discussed later) excluded patients with diastolic below 90 mmHg. Second, atenolol was used as first choice treatment with around 40% on atenolol alone at the end of year 1 though this had fallen to 20% by year 5. Other studies had thiazide as the only or one of the first line treatments. A subgroup analysis related to the first point showed a trend towards a reduction in cardiovascular disease on treatment only in patients with raised diastolic pressure. The trend in those with low diastolic pressures was towards an increase in cardiovascular disease though this was not significant. Another difference in comparison with the EWPHE study is that about one third of the EWPHE patients had a cardiovascular complication at entry. This suggests a higher risk population in EWPHE, which is thus more likely to show a benefit from treatment.

In terms of adverse effects, there was no difference in the mean score between treatment and control groups. In particular there was no difference in the risk of headache, tiredness, breathlessness, dizziness or depression. However, around 25% of patients had been unable to tolerate atenolol because of side effects such as fatigue, muscle weakness and exertional dyspnoea. Gout was reported in 11 treated patients (two controls). Diabetes mellitus developed in six treated and six control patients during the study. Biochemical testing of blood showed small but significant increases in mean concentrations of urea, creatinine, glucose and uric acid. Interestingly, despite the propaganda against thiazides and beta-blockers because of effects on lipids, there was no difference in total cholesterol between control and treated groups. Also, there was no important difference in potassium concentrations between the two groups, confirming that the vast majority of patients on low dose thiazide diuretics do not require routine potassium supplements or potassium-sparing diuretics. On balance, the authors feel that the reduction in stroke with no major problem with adverse effects justifies treatment at least up to the age of 80 when the diastolic pressure is greater than

90 mmHg. This makes systematic screening of the elderly population worthwhile. However, the 25% drop-out rate on atenolol suggests that a thiazide would be a better first choice drug.

Morbidity and mortality in the Swedish trial in old patients with hypertension (STOP-Hypertension)

One criticism of the previous studies was the use of the age of 60 as the starting point for being 'elderly' and inclusion of relatively few patients over the age of 75. This study was the first to look at a more elderly group of patients but still excluded those over the age of 84. STOP-Hypertension was a prospective, randomised, double-blind, intervention study in 1627 patients aged 70–84 years (Dahlof *et al.*, 1991).

Blood pressure was measured by the same observer for each patient throughout the study using a standard mercury sphygmomanometer. This is in contrast to the previous studies which used random zero devices and is of note in view of criticism of the accuracy of such devices (Conroy *et al.*, 1993). Pressures were measured (Korotkoff phase 5) after 5 min lying and 1 min standing using a standard cuff (12 × 35 cm) if the arm circumference was 22–32 cm. Larger or smaller cuffs were used as necessary.

A pilot study was carried out in 1985–86 with the main study carrying on from there. This multicentre study involved 116 of Sweden's 846 health centres. Untreated hypertensives were included after 1 month on placebo if blood pressure was greater than 150 mmHg systolic and 90 diastolic or diastolic above 105 on three separate occasions. Previously treated hypertensives were similarly included but had a 1–6 month washout before the placebo run-in. The main exclusions were blood pressure above 230 systolic or 120 diastolic; myocardial infarction or stroke during the past year; angina requiring drugs other than glyceryl trinitrate; and other severe incapacitating illness. A total of 812 patients were randomised to active treatment and 815 to placebo. Initial treatment was with hydrochlorothiazide 25 mg plus amiloride 2.5 mg or one of three beta-blockers (atenolol 50 mg, metoprolol 100 mg, pindolol 5 mg) once daily. Target blood pressure was 160/95 and if this had not been achieved after at least 2 months of treatment beta-blocker was added to diuretic or vice versa. If supine blood pressure was above 230/120 mmHg the patient was changed to open anti-hypertensive treatment. After a non-fatal endpoint the patient could remain on double-blind treatment.

Primary endpoints were stroke, myocardial infarction and other cardiovascular death with set criteria for defining the endpoints evaluated by an independent endpoint committee. Analysis was on an intention to treat basis using the first endpoint to occur in an individual patient. If the first endpoint was not fatal, a later fatal endpoint was included in the analysis of mortality. This occurred in 14 patients. Study power calculations suggested that 6000 patient-years would be necessary to show a significant reduction in primary endpoints, assuming that 30% of strokes and myocardial infarctions would be fatal, with a risk reduction of 1.75% per mmHg fall in systolic blood pressure and a fall in systolic pressure of 20 mmHg on active treatment compared to placebo. Recruitment took place over 5 years with the study terminating 6 months after final recruitment. Average follow-up time was 25 months. A major achievement in this study was that no patients were lost to follow-up.

The target difference of 20 mmHg in systolic blood pressure between active treatment and placebo was achieved with supine blood pressure being 19.5/8.1 mmHg lower in the active group. However, the study was stopped after only 3400 patient-years of treatment. Active treatment significantly reduced the number of primary endpoints from 94 to 58 and stroke morbidity and mortality from 53 to 29 events. Although it was not one of the primary endpoints, a significant reduction in total mortality was also observed – 63 deaths on placebo compared with 36 on active treatment.

The results obtained in this study are broadly comparable with other published figures. However, the percentage reductions observed were at the top end of the range for the major trials with 38% reduction in non-fatal stroke, 73% reduction in fatal stroke and 47% reduction in all strokes. There was a 40% reduction in all cardiovascular events but, as in most other studies, the fall in cardiac events was smaller and did not achieve statistical significance. While it is understandable that the trial was stopped because of the very convincing benefits in terms of stroke reduction, it may be that the original calculation of 6000 patient-years of treatment would have been necessary to establish a definite effect on cardiac events.

In addition to the primary endpoints, 172 secondary endpoints occurred with a clear difference between active (40 events) and placebo (132 events). The main benefits of treatment in terms of secondary endpoints were a reduction in congestive cardiac failure (39 placebo vs 19 active) and severe hypertension (75 vs 10). There was no difference in the frequency of angina (nine vs eight). The beneficial effects of active intervention were seen as early as 1 year of treatment with increasing benefit over the next 2 years. The benefits also seemed to occur at all ages in the study group.

The results from this study are thus more clear cut than in previous studies and in particular this was the first study in elderly hypertensives to show a clear benefit in terms of overall mortality. The 43% reduction in total mortality was highly significant. Are there lessons to be learned in terms of study design from the STOP trial in comparison with previous studies? It seems that there are two major differences between STOP and previous studies. First, the population was a truly elderly one with an age range of 70–84 years and an average age of 75.7 years (57% were over 75). Second, patient selection seems to have been better in the STOP trial. Although blood pressure entry criteria and the average blood pressure on entry was broadly similar between the studies, there was evidence of a more definitely hypertensive population in the STOP study if placebo blood pressures are compared (Table 4.2). Both systolic and diastolic pressures were higher than in previous studies. In view of the lower average pressures on placebo in other studies it is likely that many patients included in these studies did not have sustained hypertension. Such patients may be at lower risk of cardiovascular events and thus dilute the impact of active intervention. A further point of difference was the complete follow-up achieved in the STOP trial.

This study provides clear evidence of benefit from treatment of hypertension at least up to the age of 84 years. The absolute benefit from antihypertensive medication was that 14 elderly patients treated for 5 years would prevent one

Table 4.2 Summary of trial design criteria and blood pressures observed in six studies of hypertension in the elderly

	AUSTRAL	C&W	EWPHE	STOP	MRC	SHEP
No. of patients	582	884	840	1627	4396	4736
Age	60–69	60–79	60–97	70–84	65–74	>60
BP entry:						
systolic	<200	>170	160–239	180–230	160–209	160–219
diastolic	95–109	or >105	90–119	90–120	<115	<90
BP goal:						
systolic	–	<170	–	<160	<160	<160
diastolic	<80	<105	<90	95	–	–
Treatment						
first:	chlort	aten	hct+tri	hct+ami or beta	hct+ami or aten	chlort
add on:	various	bend	md	beta or diuret	beta or diuret	aten
BP entry	165/101	196/99	182/101	195/102	185/91	170/77
BP obtained:						
active	143/87	162/78	149/85	167/87	152/79	144/68
placebo	155/94	180/89	172/94	186/96	167/85	155/71

Drug code: ami, amiloride; aten, atenolol; bend, bendrofluazide; beta, beta-blockers; chlort, chlorthalidone; diuret, diuretic; hct, hydrochlorothiazide; md, methyldopa; tri, triamterene. References as for Table 4.1.

stroke and one death. The treatment was generally well tolerated with 58 patients on active treatment and 47 on placebo being withdrawn because of subjective side effects. This difference was not significant. In comparison with other trials the larger benefits suggest that it is worthwhile ensuring a diagnosis of sustained hypertension before starting treatment. The large numbers of patients with normal blood pressure on placebo under trial conditions suggests that many more in routine practice will be treated without good evidence of sustained hypertension. There is of course evidence from other sources (such as ambulatory monitoring – Chapter 6) to support this.

Medical Research Council trial of treatment of hypertension in older adults: principal results (MRC Working Party, 1992)

The Medical Research Council's mild hypertension trial in younger adults (aged 35–64) was begun as a pilot study in 1974 with the full trial started in 1977 and published in 1985 (MRC Working Party, 1985). This study had established a national (UK) network of collaborating general practices. The present MRC study in elderly patients was set up in 1981 using the previously established network as the basis for the trial. Recruitment took place over 5 years from March 1982. Like the Coope and Warrender (1986) study a large screening exercise was undertaken. This involved 226 group practices. A total of 184 653 invitations were sent with 125 861 (68%) attending. The age range of 65–74 was selected to follow on from the earlier study.

Blood pressure (diastolic phase 5) was measured using a Hawksley random zero sphygmomanometer. Three sitting blood pressure measurements were made with entry determined by the mean of the second and third readings being systolic 160–209 mmHg and diastolic less than 115 mmHg. Three run-in visits were made over 8 weeks by a clinic nurse – 20 389 (16% of those attending for screening) were suitable for the run-in. If the blood pressure satisfied the entry criteria, patients (8832) had it checked by a doctor. Entry to the trial was based on the doctor recording a mean blood pressure within the entry criteria, and 4961 patients were suitable. Main exclusions were treated hypertension, cardiac failure, angina, myocardial infarction or stroke within 3 months, renal impairment, diabetes, asthma or serious intercurrent disease. In total 4396 patients (3.5% of those screened) entered the randomised study.

The trial was single-blind, with the patients not knowing which treatment group they were in. Randomisation was in stratified blocks of eight to one of four treatment categories – diuretic (hydrochlorothiazide + amiloride), matching placebo, atenolol, and matching placebo. After 1985 all patients were on low dose diuretic (25 mg hydrochlorothiazide with 2.5 mg amiloride) once daily but before then higher doses had been used for some patients. Initial dose of atenolol was 50 mg once daily. A target systolic blood pressure was set for each patient – 150 mmHg if systolic <180 after run-in; 160 mmHg if >180 after run-in. Drug treatment was modified if blood pressure had not responded in 12 weeks or if target had not been achieved in 6 months. The most frequent change (225 patients) was to increase the dose of atenolol to 100 mg. For further control, atenolol could be added to diuretic and vice versa. As third-line treatment, nifedipine up to 20 mg daily or other drugs could be used. If blood pressure was sustained above systolic 210 or diastolic 115 then treatment was arranged outside the protocol and placebo patients (11%) were started on active treatment.

The main terminating events were stroke, myocardial infarction, other cardiovascular events and deaths from any cause. Diagnostic evidence for each terminating event was reviewed by an arbitrator, blinded as to the treatment regimen. If a patient had a non-fatal event followed by a fatal one in the same category only the fatal one was included in the analysis. If two different events (e.g. stroke and coronary) occurred, both were included (13 patients).

This study was designed to be larger than those previously published. It was estimated that 5000 patients would need to be followed up for 5 years to detect a 30% reduction in stroke with a power of 90% and a significance level of 2%. In reality, almost 4400 patients were followed for an average of 5.8 years, which gives 25 500 patient-years of treatment against the estimated 25 000 patient-years. As in previous studies the main analysis was on an intention to treat basis. The two placebo groups were combined.

Treatment lowered blood pressure on average only 15/6 mmHg compared to placebo with both groups showing a significant fall from entry blood pressure (Table 4.2). The 25% (95% CI 3–42%) reduction in stroke and 17% (95% CI 2–29%) reduction in all cardiovascular events was smaller than that observed for other studies and may reflect a population with lower risk. The 19% reduction in coronary events was not statistically significant. In particular, comparison with the STOP study reveals a smaller difference in blood pressure between active and placebo treatment and the placebo mean blood pressure in the Medical Research Council trial is almost identical to the active treated group in the STOP study. The age difference between STOP and Medical Research Council is also important. The design of the MRC study allowed for a separation of the diuretic and beta-blocker effects. This is particularly interesting because similar falls in blood pressure were achieved but the outcome results were quite different. The diuretic group, after adjusting for baseline characteristics, had a 31% (95% CI 3–51%) reduction in stroke, 44% (CI 21–60%) reduction in coronary events and 35% (CI 17–49%) reduction in all cardiovascular events. In contrast, there were no significant reductions for any of these endpoints in the beta-blocker group. Most of the reduction in strokes in the diuretic group occurred in non-smokers. More patients randomised to atenolol required supplementary treatment than those randomised to diuretic (52% vs 38% at 5 years).

The doctors' blood pressure measurements were on average 10/3 higher than the nurse recordings on run-in. This is in keeping with previous evidence of the adverse effect doctors have on measurement of blood pressure in some patients (Pickering *et al.*, 1988). The nurse recordings may be closer to the patient's true blood pressure. The study design did require both nurse and doctor pressures to be within a defined range but there has still been a large fall in pressure on placebo in many patients.

In comparison with other studies there was a large number of patients (25%) lost to follow-up though the cause of death was identified in all patients. There was also a higher drop-out rate due to adverse effects than in the STOP trial. These were the well-known adverse effects such as glucose intolerance, gout and muscle cramps on diuretic and Raynaud's, breathlessness and lethargy on atenolol. The beta-blocker group had a higher number of withdrawals than the diuretic group due to adverse effects. Total numbers of withdrawals for adverse effects were 160 diuretic, 333 atenolol and 82 placebo. Inadequate control of blood pressure resulted in withdrawal of one diuretic, 12 atenolol and 175 placebo patients. It is not stated whether most of the diuretic withdrawals occurred when the higher doses were used initially.

While this study was not primarily one of the treatment of isolated systolic hypertension, 43% of randomised patients had a systolic above 160 mmHg and a diastolic pressure below 90 mmHg. The patients are thus a mixture of mixed systolic/diastolic hypertension and isolated systolic hypertension in keeping with the patients seen in routine practice.

As with previous studies, the benefit for treating hypertension has been confirmed at least for diuretics and perhaps only in non-smokers. The main limitation in applying the results is the limited age range chosen for study. This is of particular concern in the UK because the upper age of this study at 75 is the age above which annual screening of blood pressure is supposed to be carried out by general practitioners.

Prevention of stroke by antihypertensive drug treatment in older persons with isolated systolic hypertension. Final results of the Systolic Hypertension in the Elderly Program (SHEP)

This is the only published trial to date which has looked exclusively at isolated systolic hypertension (ISH) (SHEP Cooperative Research Group, 1991). ISH is very much a condition affecting older patients and as such the study could not have been performed in a younger age group. SHEP was a double-blind, randomised, placebo-controlled trial in patients of 60 years old and above. Recruitment was carried out at 16 clinical centres throughout the USA from March 1985 to January 1988. In this relatively short time, an incredible 447 921 individuals were identified and contacted. Of these, 11.6% met initial criteria but only 2.7% (12094) completed baseline visit one.

Blood pressure was measured by trained technicians using Hawksley random-zero sphygmomanometers with phase five for diastolic pressure. Inclusion was on the basis of four seated blood pressure measurements at two visits being between 160 and 219 mmHg systolic and less than 90 mmHg diastolic. The main exclusions were major cardiovascular disease or other major illness such as cancer or renal failure. Randomisation took place after the second baseline visit with a total of 4736 patients being randomised (2365 active, 2371 placebo). Of this total, 3161 were previously untreated and 1575 underwent drug withdrawal before inclusion. Thus only about 1% of those initially contacted were suitable for inclusion though 90% of ineligible patients were excluded because of failure to meet the blood pressure criteria.

Active treatment was carried out by a stepped care approach. Treatment was adjusted to achieve a target systolic pressure of less than 160 mmHg if baseline was above 180 mmHg or a reduction of at least 20 mmHg if baseline systolic was 160–179 mmHg. Step one was chlorthalidone 12.5 mg daily with dose increased to 25 mg if necessary. Step two was atenolol 25 mg daily with increase to 50 mg if necessary (reserpine if atenolol was contra-indicated).

The primary endpoint was total stroke. Secondary endpoints were cardiovascular and coronary morbidity and mortality, all cause mortality and quality of life measures. Occurrence of events was confirmed by a coding panel blinded to the patients' treatment and using set criteria. The calculated sample size was 4800 participants to detect a difference of at least 32% in total stroke with 90% power at the 5% level of significance. Analysis was again on an intention to treat basis.

Although there was no upper age limit, the SHEP study had a relatively low average age of 72 years. This is similar to the EWPHE study and probably reflects either some reluctance to include very elderly patients in clinical trials or more difficulty in contacting the very elderly. The SHEP study did screen a vast number of patients but it is not clear whether the very elderly were less likely to come forward for consideration for entry to the trial. Also figures for the relative numbers of very elderly patients in these populations is not given. The SHEP patients were relatively high risk as suggested by 61% having an ECG abnormality.

Blood pressure at entry was not particularly high at a mean of 170/77. This showed a further fall in both active and placebo groups (Table 4.2) with a mean difference of 11/3 between active and placebo. At the 5 year visit, 30% of the active group were on step one low dose medication only and 16% on step one higher dose, i.e. almost 50% on thiazide alone; 23% were on step two medication but 21% were receiving additional drugs and 9% no medication. In the placebo group, active antihypertensive medication-taking increased throughout the study from 13% at year 1 to 44% at year 5. The goal blood pressure was achieved by about 70% in the active group and 36% of the placebo group.

The primary endpoint of total stroke showed a 36% reduction from 159 in the placebo group to 103 in the active group. This gave a relative risk of 0.64 (95% CI 0.50–0.82). There were also significant reductions in cardiac events (27%) and all cardiovascular events (32%). SHEP is the only study to have shown a significant reduction in all cardiac events, for example the relative risk (95% CI) for coronary heart disease was 0.75 (0.60–0.94) and non-fatal myocardial infarction 0.67 (0.47–0.96). These results are remarkable in that the reduction in blood pressure by active treatment was relatively small and the placebo group blood pressures were mainly in what we would consider as the normal range. Part of the explanation for this was the increasing number of placebo group patients started on treatment as the trial progressed.

The absolute benefit was one event prevented for 33 patients treated for 5 years. This is less convincing than the STOP results and can be explained by the differences in blood pressure between the two trials and the fact that many placebo patients in SHEP were on treatment. The true absolute benefit should thus be even more than claimed. The drugs were generally well tolerated with only small differences in adverse effects between placebo and active treatment. As in previous studies there was no major problem with metabolic effects for the vast majority of patients. As expected, there was a rise in glucose but this was little above the rise in the placebo group over 5 years. This study did not use a routine potassium sparing agent and confirmed that it is not necessary for the majority of patients.

There are reservations about the SHEP study regarding the routine treatment of ISH. First, the low blood pressures would not previously have been treated and yet clear benefit is shown in spite of the difficulties discussed above. Second, the type of patient with ISH seen in routine hospital practice tends to have much higher sustained systolic pressures (190–230 mmHg) than in SHEP. Anecdotally, these do not appear to respond well to treatment if a true diagnosis of sustained ISH can be made. This seems to apply to all drugs whether used alone or in combination. This is an area where much more research is required with other studies such as SYSTEUR ongoing (Amery *et al.*, 1991). At present it would seem sensible to treat ISH with low dose thiazide and other drugs if the blood pressure responds. In patients with failure of the blood pressure to respond to multiple drug treatment, can we do any better than treat with low dose thiazide alone? This is of particular concern in the very elderly, as will be discussed later.

Drug treatment of hypertension in the elderly. Meta-analysis of outcome trials in elderly hypertensives

This study identified 11 randomised trials of antihypertensive treatment, which were exclusively or had included elderly (over 60) patients, published between

1964 and 1992 (Thijs *et al.*, 1994). The meta-analysis concentrated on patients with systolic and diastolic hypertension and excluded three studies that did not meet pre-specified criteria – SHEP, which was isolated systolic hypertension, one that gave no absolute figures for morbidity and mortality and a third that did not compare active treatment with no treatment or placebo. The eight remaining studies were the five discussed above plus the US Veterans Administration Study Group (VACS) (1972), Hypertension-Stroke Cooperative Study Group (HSCS) (1974) and the Japanese study of mild hypertension in the aged (Kuramoto *et al.*, 1981). The combined analysis included 8701 patients (4395 active, 4306 controls), which was mainly made up of the five trials already considered (8329 patients). The other trials were small with 81 (VACS), 200 (HSCS) and 91 (Japanese) patients. Around half of the total is from the British Medical Research Council study (MRC Working Party, 1992). Five of the studies were double-blind, two single-blind and one open.

The difference in risk of experiencing a fatal event in the control group varied widely among the different trials. The authors comment on the differences in selection and recruitment (e.g. population screening, out-patient clinics) and entry criteria for blood pressure, target blood pressure and treatment used as discussed previously.

All-cause mortality showed a tendency to a small decrease (9%) but was not statistically significant (95% CI −18% to 1%). Only the STOP trial showed a really significant reduction in all-cause mortality. Non-cardiovascular mortality did not change significantly in any of the individual trials or in the meta-analysis. Overall cardiovascular mortality was lower in the active treatment group in all studies except the Japanese one with the combined analysis showing a reduction of 22% (95% CI −32% to −10%). Coronary mortality was also significantly reduced by 26% (95% CI −40% to −9%)in the pooled data. Since cerebrovascular mortality was reduced in the intervention group in the four largest studies the combined results show a significant decrease of 33% (95% CI −50% to −9%).

When non-fatal events are considered there is wide variation between the trials in the results obtained and the way the different events are defined. For example, cerebrovascular events include completed stroke but may also include transient ischaemic attacks and reversible ischaemic neurological deficits. There are similar differences in events considered as coronary. The authors felt that these differences were too great to allow a meaningful meta-analysis to be performed.

Although there is uncertainty as to reduction in all-cause mortality and some non-fatal events, it is clear that fatal cardiovascular complications are reduced. This alone forms solid evidence to justify drug treatment. It should, however, be balanced against the risks of adverse effects that have not been studied in an ideal way since the primary aim of all the trials was to determine the effects on cardiovascular outcome rather than side effects.

Most of the studies used doses of thiazide diuretic greater than is current practice. The risk of side effects with low dose thiazide is reduced (Carlsen *et al.*, 1990) and in particular metabolic effects are minimal. The adverse effects of larger dose thiazide and beta-blockers are well known but if patients can tolerate these there is no problem. The difficulty arises with patients who experience adverse effects with well-tried agents such as thiazides and beta-blockers. Should they be treated with newer drugs that they can tolerate but which have not yet been proven to reduce morbidity and mortality? The vast majority of reviews and published opinion say yes, though it should be stressed that low dose thiazide is very well tolerated and likely to be suitable first-line therapy for almost all elderly hypertensive patients.

INTERMEDIATE ENDPOINTS

It obviously takes time to evaluate new antihypertensive drugs in terms of their effect on morbidity and mortality. However, the STOP-Hypertension study (Dahlof *et al.*, 1991) has clearly shown that if elderly patients with established hypertension are properly selected it is possible to conduct a study in a reasonable number of patients with relatively short (2 years) follow-up and complete the study in 5 years. Drugs such as captopril, enalapril and nifedipine have been around for long enough for such trials to have been completed if the pharmaceutical companies producing these drugs had been prepared to fund the studies at an earlier time. Some studies are ongoing at present but it is likely to be another 2–3 years before we have published evidence of the effects of any of the newer drugs on cardiovascular events.

There is a considerable body of evidence of the effect of these drugs on lowering blood pressure and on various cardiovascular parameters. Some of these have been linked with risk of hypertensive complications such as stroke or myocardial infarction and used to support claims that such drugs will be beneficial in the treatment of hypertension. Most of the work has been linked to left ventricular hypertrophy (LVH) but relatively little has been done in elderly populations.

LEFT VENTRICULAR HYPERTROPHY

A meta-analysis of 109 treatment studies on the reversal of LVH in hypertensive patients has been published (Dahlof *et al.*, 1992). The authors only included studies that had used echocardiography to measure LVH. This is important since the sensitivity using echocardiography is close to 100% compared with only 20–50% using electrocardiographic methods. Left ventricular mass measurements are a good predictor of increased cardiovascular risk (Levy *et al.*, 1990). This is probably due to several mechanisms such as loss of cardiac reserve, accelerated atherosclerosis and arrhythmias (Frohlich, 1987). The 109 studies included 2357 patients with an average age of 49 years (range 30–71). The results of this analysis are thus of little relevance to elderly patients but are a useful guide for comparing the results from studies in an elderly population. One other obvious problem is that the studies are mainly very small with an average number of 22 patients (range 4–70) per study. Only three of the studies were randomised, double-blind in previously untreated patients. Most (80; 73%) were open and uncontrolled.

Overall left ventricular mass (LVM) was reduced by 11.9% (95% CI 10.1–13.7) for a 14.9% (14–15.8) reduction in mean arterial pressure. The authors then adjusted for differences between studies to allow comparison between different drug groups. The results are shown in Table 4.3.

Table 4.3   Reduction of LVM with different drug groups

Drug group	Reduction in LVM % (95% CI)	Absolute reduction (g)
ACE inhibitors	15.0 (9.9–20.1)	44.7
Beta-blockers	8.0 (4.8–11.2)	22.8
Calcium antagonists	8.5 (5.1–11.8)	26.9
Diuretics	11.3 (5.6–17)	21.4

The authors conclude that ACE inhibitors are the most effective at reducing LVM by reversing wall hypertrophy but beta-blockers and calcium antagonists also do this to a lesser extent. In contrast, diuretics mainly reduce ventricular diameter. They also state that the prognostic implications need to be evaluated in a controlled prospective trial.

Only three of the studies (Frishman *et al.*, 1989; Schulman *et al.*, 1990; Vyssoulis *et al.*, 1990) contained elderly patients but these were relatively young elderly. In one study in elderly patients atenolol had no effect on LVH regression whereas verapamil did reduce LVM by 18% (Schulman *et al.*, 1990). Unfortunately there is no other data to support or refute this finding in elderly patients.

Left ventricular mass increases with age independent of blood pressure (Levy *et al.*, 1989). In hypertensive elderly patients, the prevalence of LVH may be over 50% (Aronow *et al.*, 1991; Jones *et al.*, 1990). A recent study (James *et al.*, 1994) has examined the prevalence of LVH in relation to ambulatory and clinic blood pressures in 52 elderly hypertensive patients with a mean age of 76 years (range 63–87). About half of the patients were previously untreated and all were off treatment at the time of the study. Left ventricular mass index (LVMI) was calculated (LVM divided by body surface area) and 83% of the subjects found to have LVH taking LVMI as greater than $135 \, g/m^2$ for men or $110 \, g/m^2$ for women. LVMI showed relatively weak ($r < 0.3$) correlations with clinic systolic blood pressure, ambulatory daytime systolic BP and night-time diastolic BP. There was a stronger correlation ($r = 0.41$) between LVMI and night-time systolic BP. Also patients with a bigger difference (>10 mmHg) between day and night systolic BP had significantly lower LVMI values. The importance of ambulatory blood pressure monitoring is considered in detail in Chapter 6. The conclusion from this study is that night-time blood pressures are most closely correlated to LVH. The study emphasises the importance of the nocturnal dip in reducing overall blood pressure load.

The effect of antihypertensives on other ECG parameters has also been claimed to be a useful guide to choice of individual drug. A study of bendrofluazide and captopril was carried out in 80 untreated hypertensive patients with mild cognitive impairment identified from a community screening programme (Starr and Whalley, 1993). Patients with existing heart disease were excluded but there was still a high prevalence (35%) of ECG abnormalities on screening. The fall in blood pressure was similar for both drugs but the captopril group showed a reduction in overall ECG abnormalities and a significant reduction in QRS duration from 0.8 to 0.7 seconds. The bendrofluazide group showed the same fall in QRS but this was not statistically significant. The authors claim that their results support the use of captopril as an alternative to bendrofluazide but the evidence is not entirely convincing and further study is required.

All of the studies of drug effects in LVH have looked at whether or not regression of existing LVH occurs with treatment. Whilst this is important, consideration needs to be given as to whether drugs might behave differently in terms of preventing the development of LVH in patients who do not have ventricular hypertrophy at the start of treatment. The major outcome studies discussed above all carried out ECGs on the patients at baseline and during the study. However, none of the studies used LVH as an outcome measure and the results are not readily available. Even if the results were known, they would still have to be treated with caution because of the well-recognised poor sensitivity of the ECG as a measure of LVH. A study using echocardiography may well be impractical because of the numbers of patients necessary.

EFFECTS ON OTHER CARDIOVASCULAR DISEASES

Although not directly related to outcome in the treatment of hypertension it is worthwhile considering the benefits of antihypertensive drugs in other cardiovascular diseases. Both ACE inhibitors and calcium channel antagonists have been studied, although most of the reports are of the benefits of various ACE inhibitors in patients with cardiac failure. The studies have not specifically looked at elderly patients but have included patients up to the 'younger' elderly age group.

The first study to show benefit in terms of survival on angiotensin-converting enzyme inhibitors (ACE inhibitors) in cardiac failure was published in 1987 (Consensus Trial Study Group, 1987). This trial included 253 patients with severe congestive heart failure (NYHA class IV) and a mean age of 70 years. A significant ($P = 0.003$) 27% reduction in mortality (68 deaths on placebo, 50 on enalapril) was observed. Improvement in NYHA classification, reduction in heart size and reduced requirement for other heart failure medication were also recorded.

Four years later, further evidence of benefit in patients with less severe cardiac failure was published (SOLVD Investigators, 1991). The SOLVD study recruited 2569 patients with a mean age of 61 years. All had chronic heart failure with an ejection fraction of less than 0.35. About 90% were NYHA class II and III. Again, a significant reduction in mortality was noted in the enalapril treated group. The reduction in risk was 16% (95% CI 5–26%) based on 510 deaths (39.7%) in the placebo group and 452 (35.2%) in the enalapril group. The largest reduction was in death due to progressive cardiac failure. The SOLVD investigators also studied the effects of enalapril in asymptomatic patients with known heart disease and ejection fractions less than 0.35 (SOLVD Investigators, 1992). This study showed a significant reduction in the incidence of heart failure and rate of hospitalisation with enalapril. There was also a trend towards a reduction (8%) in risk of death but this was not statistically significant.

Other ACE inhibitors have also been studied and recent publications have concentrated on post-myocardial infarction patients. Captopril was used in the

SAVE study (1992) of 2231 post-myocardial infarction patients with a left ventricular ejection fraction of less than 40% and no overt heart failure. A 21% reduction in cardiovascular mortality was observed, with reductions in the development of heart failure (36%) and hospitalisation due to heart failure (22%). The AIRE study (2006 patients, mean age 65 years) used ramipril in post-myocardial infarction patients with clinical evidence of heart failure (Acute Infarction Ramipril Efficacy (AIRE) Study Investigators, 1993). A risk reduction of 27% (95% CI 11–40%) was observed based on 222 deaths on placebo and 170 on ramipril. Lisinopril also produced a significant reduction in overall mortality (odds ratio 0.88; 95% CI 0.79–0.99) in post-myocardial infarction patients (Gruppo Italiano per lo Studio della Sopravvivenza nell Infarto Miocardico, 1994).

There is therefore clear evidence of benefit from the use of ACE inhibitors in patients with cardiac failure and after myocardial infarction. However, the benefit was least in patients without symptoms of cardiac failure when the small reduction in mortality was not statistically significant (SOLVD Investigators, 1992). The benefits cannot therefore be directly extrapolated to the treatment of hypertension though many patients with hypertension will develop left ventricular failure. The evidence is not enough to justify use of an ACE inhibitor as first-line treatment if a patient is suitable for a thiazide diuretic. However, when a second drug is required the available evidence favours an ACE inhibitor over alternatives such as a calcium channel blocker or alpha-blocker. Ongoing trials should resolve this dilemma in the near future.

The case for using calcium channel blockers is far less convincing. An overview of 28 randomised trials of the use of calcium channel blockers in myocardial infarction and angina found no evidence of a reduction in risk of death or of the risk of initial or recurrent myocardial infarction (Held *et al.*, 1989). Most of the studies had used nifedipine with less use of other agents such as verapamil or diltiazem. In the Danish study of verapamil in myocardial infarction 1775 patients were recruited, with 609 being over the age of 65 years (Danish Study Group on Verapamil in Myocardial Infarction, 1990). A significant reduction in mortality (7.7% in verapamil group, 11.8% placebo) was found in the patients without heart failure but there was no difference in mortality in the patients with heart failure. Age did not influence these results. The debate concerning deleterious effects of short-acting calcium blockers in both post-infarction and hypertension are discussed in Chapter 5. Therefore, it is difficult to justify the widespread use of nifedipine as first-line treatment for hypertension until evidence of benefit is produced.

EFFECTS ON BLOOD PRESSURE

Only small numbers of patients are required to show whether or not a drug lowers blood pressure. However, great care is necessary in designing and carrying out the study to avoid the tendency for blood pressure to fall with time being confused with a genuine drug effect. The large multicentre studies have demonstrated the extent of fall in blood pressure with time and placebo even after the run-in phase. For example, mean falls of 16/10, 10/7, 9/6 and 18/6 mmHg were recorded in the Coope and Warrender, EWPHE, STOP-Hypertension and MRC elderly trials respectively (Coope and Warrender, 1986; Amery *et al.*, 1985; Dahlof *et al.*, 1991; MRC Working Party, 1992).

An enormous number of comparative studies of different antihypertensive drugs have been performed though very few in elderly patients. The results are often conflicting and it is not proposed to discuss many of those studies. Two studies have compared a wide range of drugs and these are most useful as a starting point for determining the relative efficacy of different antihypertensive agents.

Treatment of mild hypertension study

This study will eventually publish data on morbidity and mortality but the initial results comparing non-pharmacological treatment with five different drugs on blood pressure over one year have been published (Treatment of Mild Hypertension Research Group, 1991). A total of 902 patients were randomised into this double-blind, placebo-controlled study. This gives a sound data base for comparing different drugs in terms of effect on blood pressure, but is relatively small for looking at morbidity and mortality effects. All participants received non-pharmacological intervention in the form of weight reduction if necessary, fat modified diet, reduced dietary sodium, reduced alcohol intake and increased leisure-time activity. There were approximately 130 patients in each of the five drug treatment groups and 234 in the placebo group. The patients were aged 45–69 years (mean 55) and had mild hypertension as defined by diastolic BP 90–99 mmHg over three eligibility visits. All drugs were given once daily in the following doses – chlorthalidone 15 mg, acebutolol 400 mg, doxazosin 2 mg, amlodipine 5 mg and enalapril 5 mg. If necessary, a second drug was added – chlorthalidone 15 mg in all cases except the diuretic group who received enalapril as the second drug. A random zero sphygmomanometer was used with cuff size depending on the size of the patient's arm. The blood pressure reductions from baseline are noted in Table 4.4.

Table 4.4 Blood pressure reductions (mmHg)

Blood pressure	Acebutolol	Amlodipine	Chlorthalidone	Doxazosin	Enalapril	Placebo
Systolic	20.1	17.5	21.8	16.1	17.6	10.6
Diastolic	13.7	12.9	13.1	12.0	12.2	8.1

All the drugs were significantly better than placebo. Between-drug comparisons showed a significant difference only in systolic pressure between chlorthalidone and doxazosin. All five groups of drugs thus had similar antihypertensive effects in patients with mild hypertension. Only 17% of patients required a second drug. The doses of enalapril and doxazosin were lower than usually prescribed and this study does not show the maximum possible reduction in blood pressure with each type of drug. Nevertheless it does give some evidence that there is little to choose between the different types of agent in terms of blood pressure reduction. Also, in this study there was little difference between the drugs in terms of safety, tolerability and impact on quality of life.

Single drug therapy for hypertension in men

This was another large, randomised, double-blind study involving 1292 men (Materson *et al.*, 1993). As in the TOMHS study the five main classes of drug were compared with placebo but in addition clonidine was included. The main differences between the two studies are the obvious one of no females in this study, a higher entry diastolic blood pressure of 95–109 mmHg and the doses of drugs used were titrated as necessary but were within the dose range used in routine practice.

The study looked at a younger age group (<60 years, mean age 50) of 546 patients and an older group (>60 years, mean age 66) of 746 patients. There were approximately 180 patients in each treatment group at randomisation but only 41% of patients initially randomised completed the study. Most drop outs (410) were because the patients did not meet the criteria for the maintenance phase. The daily doses of drugs used were hydrochlorothiazide 12.5–50 mg, atenolol 25–100 mg, captopril 25–100 mg, clonidine 0.2–0.6 mg, diltiazem sustained release 120–360 mg and prazosin 4–20 mg. The drug doses were titrated to achieve a diastolic pressure of less than 90 mmHg.

The average reductions in blood pressure from baseline to the end of the titration period are shown in Table 4.5.

Table 4.5 Average blood pressure reductions (mmHg)

Blood pressure	Hydrochlort	Atenolol	Captopril	Clonidine	Diltiazem	Prazosin	Placebo
Systolic	14	11	9	16	13	12	3
Diastolic	10	12	10	12	14	11	5

Diltiazem had the highest rate of success with 59% reaching the target blood pressure compared with 51% for atenolol, 50% for clonidine, 46% for hydrochlorothiazide, 42% for captopril and 42% for prazosin. There was also a tendency for differences depending on race and age. Diltiazem was best for Blacks of both age groups with 64% reaching goal blood pressure. Captopril was best for younger Whites (55%), while atenolol was best for older Whites (68%). Drug intolerance was more of a problem with clonidine and prazosin than with the other drugs.

This study does show small differences in the response to different types of antihypertensive drug but these are not big enough to seriously modify the choice of drug for different patients except for the known poor response of Black races to beta-blockers.

Although elderly patients showed a good response to atenolol there is a problem because a significant proportion of elderly patients have a contra-indication to the use of beta-blockers. In addition, we already know that thiazides are more effective than beta-blockers in reducing stroke in hypertensive elderly patients.

Comparisons of antihypertensive drugs in elderly patients

It is not proposed to comprehensively review the comparisons of different hypertensive drugs but simply to highlight a few examples.

Diltiazem has been shown to have similar response rates to hydrochlorothiazide or hydrochlorothiazide/triamterene in three studies in elderly patients. One of these included patients up to the age of 95 (mean 74) years (Djian *et al.*, 1990). In all three studies the tendency was for diltiazem to produce a higher percentage of responders (Djian *et al.*, 1990; Leehey and Hartman, 1988; Robitaille, 1991). The results were similar to the Veterans study with 50–71% responding to thiazide and 69–83% to diltiazem. A comparison of diltiazem with enalapril and atenolol in elderly women (mean age 70 years) found response rates of 77, 67 and 63%, respectively (Applegate *et al.*, 1991). There was no significant difference in response between diltiazem and enalapril, unlike the difference found between diltiazem and captopril in males in the Veterans study. Comparison with other calcium antagonists found no difference between diltiazem and isradipine (Black *et al.*, 1992) or between diltiazem, verapamil and nifedipine (Markham and Brogden, 1993).

Similarly, amlodipine, which was used in the TOMHS study, has been compared with other drugs. These have been reviewed but not specifically in elderly patients (Murdoch and Heel, 1991). In two studies, amlodipine was compared with atenolol but unlike the TOMHS study the response rate was higher for atenolol than amlodipine, although the results are broadly comparable with other studies. In a comparison with hydrochlorothiazide, amlodipine was slightly more effective with a response rate of 74% compared to 70%. The response rate to thiazide in this study was much higher than in the larger Veterans study. A comparison with verapamil showed a typical 72% response to amlodipine but only 48% to verapamil. This is in contrast with other work which suggests that different calcium antagonists have a similar effect on blood pressure.

In isolated systolic hypertension, amlodipine and enalapril were compared in 31 patients aged 45–76 years using clinic and ambulatory blood pressure recording (Webster *et al.*, 1993). Systolic blood pressure (mean) fell from 185 to 164 mmHg with amlodipine and from 183 to 159 with enalapril. There was thus no difference between the drugs for supine systolic blood pressure. In addition there was no difference in the effect on diastolic blood pressure and these clinic results were confirmed by the ambulatory recordings.

Overall there is therefore little to choose between different drugs in terms of their effects on blood pressure. Choice of initial drug should be guided by trial results using real disease endpoints. However, about half of patients may require additional treatment and the second-line drug will often have to be used without clear evidence of benefit. Since the drugs currently available are all broadly similar, the choice should depend on individual patient factors rather than possible small differences in the degree of blood pressure reduction.

Other considerations

When a drug is prescribed for 'life' we hope that most patients will achieve the desired therapeutic response and be able to tolerate it. A large general practice study of 37 643 patients with hypertension in the United Kingdom suggests that this is not the case for all four major classes of antihypertensive drugs (Jones *et al.*, 1995). Less than half of patients started on a new drug were still taking it after 6 months. There was little to choose between the different drugs. The study covered all ages with 59% over the age of 65 years. These results are different from those in controlled clinical trials but may well reflect the real situation in routine practice. The reasons for the poor rate of continuation with therapy are unclear.

A recent study of medication predisposing to falls in elderly patients found a major problem with calcium channel blockers (Koski *et al.*, 1996). The odds ratios were 3.0 for all injuries in men, 2.5 for all injuries in women and 2.4 for major injuries in women. If confirmed, this result is further evidence for not using calcium blockers as first-line treatment in elderly patients.

SHOULD VERY ELDERLY PATIENTS BE TREATED?

Patients aged over 80–84 years were specifically excluded from most of the blood pressure trials in elderly patients. The EWPHE and SHEP studies had no upper age limit but the numbers of patients over the age of 80 were relatively small. The EWPHE study had only 155 patients over 80 and thus there was insufficient power to be able to show any benefit. However, the SHEP study was able to show a 45% reduction in stroke incidence in 649 patients (Bulpitt, 1994). There is still considerable debate as to whether or not hypertension should be treated in the very elderly and if so what should be the level to initiate treatment and what target blood pressure should be aimed for.

One argument against treating is that the very elderly are survivors. High blood pressure is not a risk indicator for cardiovascular or total mortality in men over the age of 75 and women over the age of 85. There is also evidence that very elderly hypertensive patients may live longer than those with lower blood pressure. In a prospective study of 561 older people (>85 years) in one region in Finland followed up for 5 years, mortality was greatest in the group with lowest blood pressure and lowest in those with systolic pressure above 160 and diastolic above 90 mmHg (Mattila *et al.*, 1988). This relationship occurred both in patients living at home and those in institutional care. The population studied was 83% of those aged 85 or over in the Tampere region who were divided into six groups according to blood pressure. Although numbers in the extreme blood pressure groups were small it was clear that survival increased at least up to 160 mmHg systolic and 90–99 mmHg diastolic with a tendency to plateau above these levels. In a further study of 2270 people aged over 65 years in California a paradoxical increase in survival was found only in men aged over 75 years with increasing diastolic pressure (Langer *et al.*, 1989). This result is thus less convincing than the Finish study but does show we cannot simply assume that treating hypertension will be beneficial in the very old.

Elderly patients are different. Aortic compliance falls and leads to an increase in systolic pressure and a decrease in diastolic pressure. This results in many patients with isolated systolic hypertension, which has been shown to benefit from treatment (SHEP Cooperative Research Group, 1991). However, the mean level of systolic pressure in the SHEP study was well below the optimum level for survival in the very old. It is not clear whether there is benefit from treating much higher levels of isolated systolic hypertension at any age.

It is certainly possible to discuss the theoretical and epidemiological evidence in terms of whether or not to treat very elderly patients. However, only good quality clinical trial evidence of active treatment compared with placebo can really answer the question. Even though patients with higher untreated blood pressure survive longer, this does not exclude the possibility that treatment might improve survival even more. Several trials are ongoing at present, which should help resolve this problem. Two studies of isolated systolic hypertension have included a very elderly subgroup – SYSTEUR (Amery *et al.*, 1991) and SYS-CHINA (Systolic Hypertension in the Elderly Collaborative Group Coordinating Center, 1992). In addition, there is a study of patients with both diastolic and systolic hypertension exclusively in very elderly patients (HYVET – Bulpitt *et al.*, 1994).

These studies should resolve the question of whether or not to treat newly diagnosed very elderly hypertensive patients. This is particularly important since there is a tendency to screen elderly patients for hypertension in several countries. Clearly there is no point in measuring blood pressure in the over 80s unless we can give clear advice on how to manage the condition if it is diagnosed. An additional problem is what to do with a treated hypertensive patient who reaches the age of 85. Should treatment be continued at the same level, reduced or stopped? There is no clear answer to this but if the patient is tolerating the treatment it is often difficult to stop after years of encouragement to comply with medication. It is easier to maintain the status quo and continue treatment until the above studies report their results.

NEW DRUGS

Several new drugs are under development and likely to appear within the next few years. The first of the angiotensin II receptor antagonists, losartan, has recently been marketed. Losartan has been shown to be as effective as existing drugs such as captopril, atenolol and felodipine (Hansson, 1995). It also appears to be well tolerated and to cause less coughing than the ACE inhibitors. As with all new drugs, there is limited experience of its use in elderly patients and no information on the effect on morbidity and mortality.

CONCLUSIONS

There is now unequivocal evidence of benefit from treating hypertension in elderly patients. Despite differences in the study design, study population and drugs used, there is remarkable agreement in results in terms of stroke reduction. The benefits in terms of cardiac disease are less marked but nevertheless there is a tendency towards benefit in all the studies. The drugs were also very well tolerated in most patients, particularly with the trend towards using low dose thiazide diuretic as the first-line drug.

How easy is it to implement these results in routine practice? The rule of halves, which states that only half of hypertension in the community is detected, only half detected is treated and only half of that treated is well controlled, has not been formally tested by screening an elderly population. There is no reason to suspect that the reality is much different from younger age groups. A relatively recent Scottish study in patients aged 45–59 showed that little progress has been made (Smith *et al.*, 1990). In an attempt to examine this problem in an elderly population, a recent study used a random sample of general practitioner case notes (6987 patients aged 65–80) to obtain information on diagnosis of hypertension, whether treated and whether controlled (Ford *et al.*, 1996). Their findings suggested a modified rule of halves, with 25% of patients undetected, 25% of detected patients untreated and 53% of treated patients controlled. This gives an overall figure of 29% detected, treated and controlled (compared with 12.5 in rule of halves). This study clearly could not hope to look at the whole population, which is the only way of detecting all hypertension. However, population screening with a single blood pressure measurement has its own problems such as overdiagnosing true hypertension.

In terms of detection, the trend towards increased screening of elderly patients should increase awareness of the presence of hypertension to a high level. There is now no excuse for not treating hypertension in elderly patients, though care should be taken to ensure a diagnosis of sustained hypertension before starting treatment. This is an area of difficulty. Even in the clinical trials, where care was taken to ensure several blood pressure readings within the inclusion range before starting treatment, there were large numbers of patients with normal blood pressure on treatment with placebo. It is likely that more patients with 'normal' blood pressure will receive treatment in routine practice than in clinical trials. This results in patients being put at risk of adverse effects with little or no benefit from treatment. The most usual entry blood pressure in the trials was a diastolic above 90 and a systolic above 160. If these figures are interpreted too literally it will result in many patients receiving unnecessary treatment. However, if we could ensure a definite diagnosis of sustained hypertension then treatment should begin at levels above these figures. I personally tend to treat at values of 170/100 and above and regard those between 160–170 systolic and 90–100 diastolic as a grey area worthy of a period of further observation and follow-up before starting treatment. If treatment is commenced then blood pressure should be lowered to below 160/90 if it can be achieved without making the patient unwell. If drug adverse events occur with several or all the possible drug choices it becomes a fine balance between expected benefit in the longer-term and quality of life in the short-term. Only the patient can really decide what he/she prefers.

REFERENCES

Acute Infarction Ramipril Efficacy (AIRE) Study Investigators 1993. Effect of ramipril on mortality and morbidity of survivors of acute myocardial infarction with clinical evidence of heart failure. *Lancet* **342**, 821–8.
Amery A, Berthaux P, Bulpitt C *et al.* 1978. Glucose intolerance during diuretic therapy.

Results of trial by the European Working Party on hypertension in the elderly. *Lancet* **i**, 681–3.

Amery A, Birkenhager W, Bogaert M *et al.* 1982. Antihypertensive therapy in patients above age 60 with systolic hypertension. A progress report of the European Working Party on High Blood Pressure in the Elderly (EWPHE). *Clinical and Experimental Hypertension* **A4**, 1151–76.

Amery A, Birkenhager W, Brixko P *et al.* 1985. Mortality and morbidity results from the European working party on high blood pressure in the elderly trial. *Lancet* **i**, 1349–54.

Amery A, Birkenhager W, Bulpitt CJ *et al.* 1991. Syst-Eur. A multicentre trial on the treatment of isolated systolic hypertension in the elderly: objectives, protocol and organisation. *Aging* **3**, 287–302.

Applegate WB, Phillips HL, Schnaper H *et al.* 1991. A randomised controlled trial of the effects of three antihypertensive agents on blood pressure control and quality of life in older women. *Archives of Internal Medicine* **151**, 1817–23.

Aronow WS, Ahn C, Kronzon I, Koenigsberg M 1991. Congestive heart failure, coronary events and atherothrombotic brain infarction in elderly Blacks and Whites with systemic hypertension and with and without echocardiographic and electrocardiographic evidence of left ventricular hypertrophy. *American Journal of Cardiology* **67**, 295–9.

Australian Therapeutic Trial Management Committee 1980. The Australian therapeutic trial in mild hypertension. *Lancet* **i**, 1261–7.

Australian Therapeutic Trial Management Committee 1981. Treatment of mild hypertension in the elderly: a study initiated and administered by the National Heart Foundation of Australia. *Medical Journal of Australia* **ii**, 398–402.

Black HR, Lewin AJ, Stein GH *et al.* 1992. A comparison of the safety of therapeutically equivalent doses of isradipine and diltiazem for treatment of essential hypertension. *American Journal of Hypertension* **5**, 141–6.

Bulpitt CJ 1994. Hypertension in the very elderly. *Journal of Human Hypertension* **8**, 603–5.

Bulpitt CJ, Fletcher AE, Amery A *et al.* 1994. The hypertension in the very elderly trial (HYVET). *Journal of Human Hypertension* **8**, 631–2.

Carlsen JE, Kober L, Torp-Pedersen C 1990. Relation between dose of bendrofluazide, antihypertensive effect and adverse biochemical effects. *British Medical Journal* **300**, 975–8.

Conroy RM, O'Brien E, O'Malley K, Atkins N 1993. Measurement error in the Hawksley random-zero sphygmomanometer: what damage has been done and what can we learn? *British Medical Journal* **306**, 1319–22.

Consensus Trial Study Group 1987. Effects of enalapril on mortality in severe congestive heart failure. Results of the Cooperative North Scandinavian Enalapril Survival Study (Consensus). *New England Journal of Medicine* **316**, 1429–35.

Coope J 1982. A trial of treatment of hypertension in the elderly in general practice. *Acta Medica Scandinavia* **676**(Suppl.), 141–50.

Coope J, Warrender TS 1986. Randomised trial of treatment of hypertension in elderly patients in primary care. *British Medical Journal* **293**, 1145–51.

Dahlof B, Lindholm LH, Hansson L, Schersten B, Ekbom T, Wester P-O 1991. Morbidity and mortality in the Swedish trial in old patients with hypertension (STOP-Hypertension). *Lancet* **338**, 1281–5.

Dahlof B, Pennart K, Hansson L 1992. Reversal of left ventricular hypertrophy in hypertensive patients. A meta-analysis of 109 treatment studies. *American Journal of Hypertension* **5**, 95–110.

Danish Study Group on Verapamil in Myocardial Infarction 1990. Effect of verapamil on mortality and major events after acute myocardial infarction (The Danish Verapamil Infarction Trial II – DAVIT II). *American Journal of Cardiology* **66**, 779–85.

Djian J, Roy M, Forette B, Lekieffre J, Lucioni R 1990. Efficacy and tolerance of sustained-release diltiazem 300 mg and a diuretic in the elderly. *Journal of Cardiovascular Pharmacology* **16**(Suppl.), 51–5.

European Working Party on High Blood Pressure in the Elderly (EWPHE) 1985. An international trial of antihypertensive therapy in elderly patients. Objectives, protocol and organisation. *Archives International Pharmacodynamics* **275**, 300–34.

Ford GA, Duggan S, Eccles M 1996. Management of hypertension in older people in Northern Region of England. Presented at British Geriatrics Society, Canterbury, April 1996.

Frishman WH, Glasser SP, Strom JA, Schoenberger JA, Liebson P, Poland MP 1989. Effects of dilevalol, metoprolol and atenolol on left ventricular mass and function in nonelderly and elderly hypertensive patients. *American Journal of Cardiology* **63**, 69I–74I.

Frohlich ED 1987. Potential mechanisms explaining the risk of left ventricular hypertrophy. *American Journal of Cardiology* **59**, 91A–7A.

Gruppo Italiano per lo Studio della Sopravvivenza nell Infarto Miocardico 1994. GISSI–3: effects of lisinopril and transdermal glyceryl trinitrate singly and together on 6-week mortality and ventricular function after acute myocardial infarction. *Lancet* **343**, 1115–22.

Hansson L 1995. The future role of losartan. *Journal of Human Hypertension* **9**(Suppl. 5), S55–8.

Held PH, Yusuf S, Furberg CD 1989. Calcium channel blockers in acute myocardial infarction and unstable angina: an overview. *British Medical Journal* **299**, 1187–92.

Hypertension-Stroke Cooperative Study Group 1974. Effect of antihypertensive treatment on stroke recurrence. *Journal of the American Medical Association* **229**, 409–18.

James MA, Fotherby MD, Potter JF 1994. Clinical correlates of left ventricular mass in elderly hypertensives. *Journal of Human Hypertension* **8**, 409–15.

Jones E, Morgan TO, Califiore P, Johns J 1990. Prevalence of left ventricular hypertrophy in elderly patients with well controlled hypertension. *Clinical and Experimental Pharmacology and Physiology* **17**, 207–10.

Jones JK, Gorkin L, Lian JF, Staffa JA, Fletcher AP 1995. Discontinuation of and changes in treatment after start of new courses of antihypertensive drugs: a study of a United Kingdom population. *British Medical Journal* **311**, 293–5.

Kannel WB, Dawber TR 1974. Hypertension as an ingredient of a cardiovascular risk profile. *British Journal of Hospital Medicine* **11**, 508–23.

Koski K, Luukinen H, Laippala P, Kivela SL 1996. Physiological factors and medications as predictors of injurious falls by elderly people: a prospective population-based study. *Age and Ageing* **25**, 29–38.

Kuramoto K, Matsushita S, Kuwajima I, Murakawi M 1981. Prospective study on the treatment of mild hypertension in the aged. *Japanese Heart Journal* **22**, 75–85.

Langer RD, Ganiats TG, Barrett-Connor E 1989. Paradoxical survival of elderly men with high blood pressure. *British Medical Journal* **298**, 1356–8.

Leehey DJ, Hartman E 1988. Comparison of diltiazem and hydrochlorothiazide for treatment of patients 60 years of age or older with systemic hypertension. *American Journal of Cardiology* **62**, 1218–23.

Levy D, Garrison RJ, Kannel WB, Castelli WP 1990. Prognostic implications of echocardiographically determined left ventricular mass in the Framingham Heart Study. *New England Journal of Medicine* **322**, 1561–6.

Levy D, Garrison RJ, Savage DD, Kannel WB, Castelli WP 1989. Left ventricular mass and incidence of coronary heart disease in an elderly cohort. The Framingham Heart Study. *Annals of Internal Medicine* **110**, 101–7.

Markham A, Brogden RN 1993. Diltiazem. A review of its pharmacology and therapeutic use in older patients. *Drugs and Aging* **3**, 363–90.

Materson BJ, Reda DJ, Cushman WC *et al.* for the Department of Veterans Affairs Cooperative Study Group on Antihypertensive Agents 1993. Single-drug therapy for hypertension in men. A comparison of six antihypertensive agents with placebo. *New England Journal of Medicine* **328**, 914–21.

Mattila K, Haavisto M, Rajala S, Heikinheimo R 1988. Blood pressure and five year survival in the very old. *British Medical Journal* **296**, 887–9.

MRC Working Party 1985. Medical Research Council trial of treatment of mild hypertension: principal results. *British Medical Journal* **291**, 97–104.

MRC Working Party 1992. Medical Research Council trial of treatment of hypertension in older adults: principal results. *British Medical Journal* **304**, 405–12.

Murdoch D, Heel RC 1991. Amlodipine. A review of its pharmacodynamic and pharmacokinetic properties, and therapeutic use in cardiovascular disease. *Drugs* **41**, 478–505.

Pickering TG, James GD, Boddie C, Harshfield GA, Blank S, Laragh JH 1988. How common is white coat hypertension? *Journal of the American Medical Association* **259**, 225–8.

Robitaille N-M 1991. Canadian Diltiazem Study Group in the Elderly. Use of diltiazem as an antihypertensive drug in elderly. *American Journal of Hypertension* **4**, 4A.

SAVE Investigators 1992. Effect of captopril on mortality and morbidity in patients with left ventricular dysfunction after myocardial infarction. Results of the survival and ventricular enlargement trial. *New England Journal of Medicine* **327**, 669–77.

Schulman SP, Weiss JL, Becker LC *et al.* 1990. The effects of antihypertensive therapy on left ventricular mass in elderly patients. *New England Journal of Medicine* **322**, 1350–6.

SHEP Cooperative Research Group 1991. Prevention of stroke by antihypertensive drug treatment in older persons with isolated systolic hypertension. Final results of the Systolic Hypertension in the Elderly Program (SHEP). *Journal of the American Medical Association* **265**, 3255–64.

Smith WCS, Lee AJ, Crombie IK, Tunstall-Pedoe H 1990. Control of blood pressure in Scotland: the rule of halves. *British Medical Journal* **300**, 981–3.

SOLVD Investigators 1991. Effect of enalapril on survival in patients with reduced left ventricular ejection fractions and congestive heart failure. *New England Journal of Medicine* **325**, 293–302.

SOLVD Investigators 1992. Effect of enalapril on mortality and the development of heart failure in asymptomatic patients with reduced left ventricular ejection fractions. *New England Journal of Medicine* **327**, 685–91.

Starr JM, Whalley LJ 1993. Hypertensive old people in Edinburgh (HOPE) study: electrocardiographic changes after captopril or bendrofluazide treatment. *Age and Ageing* **22**, 343–8.

Systolic Hypertension in the Elderly Collaborative Group Coordinating Center 1992. Systolic hypertension in the elderly: Chinese trial (Syst-China): interim report. *Journal of Cardiology* **20**, 270–5.

Thijs L, Van Hoof R, Staessen J, Fagard R, Celis H, Amery A 1994. Drug treatment of hypertension in the elderly. In Swales JD (ed.), *Textbook of hypertension*. Oxford: Blackwell Scientific Publications, 1186–94.

Treatment of Mild Hypertension Research Group 1991. The treatment of mild hypertension study. A randomised, placebo-controlled trial of a nutritional–hygienic regimen along with various drug monotherapies. *Archives of Internal Medicine* **151**, 1413–23.

Veterans Administration Cooperative Study on Antihypertensive Agents 1972. Effects of treatment on morbidity in hypertension III. Influence of age, diastolic pressure and prior cardiovascular disease. Further analysis of side effects. *Circulation* **45**, 991–1004.

Vyssoulis G, Karpanou EA, Pitsavos CE, Paleologos AA, Kourtis TK, Toutouzas PK 1990. Left ventricular hypertrophy regression and function changes with ketanserin in elderly hypertensives. *Cardiovascular Drugs and Therapeutics* **4**, 81–4.

Webster J, Fowler G, Jeffers TA *et al.* 1993. A comparison of amlodipine with enalapril in the treatment of isolated systolic hypertension. *British Journal of Clinical Pharmacology* **35**, 499–505.

CHAPTER 5

Clinical pharmacology of antihypertensive drugs in the older adult

JOHN WEBSTER ———————————————————————

INTRODUCTION

Elevated blood pressure often merits drug treatment, and the absolute benefits from treatment are greater in the elderly than in younger patients. Patients should not be denied drug therapy simply because of advancing years. However, it is important not to extrapolate too far from data acquired in younger patients, and therapy should be guided primarily by evidence of efficacy from major outcome trials.

Some aspects of ageing are clearly important when choosing an antihypertensive drug, however:

1. The elderly are susceptible to postural hypotension, with resultant dizziness, falls or syncope. In addition they are less able to compensate for disequilibrium on account of coexistent musculoskeletal disorders.
2. The elderly frequently suffer from cardiovascular diseases such as angina, heart failure, myocardial infarction, peripheral vascular disease and arrhythmias, all of which may influence the choice of therapy. Renal insufficiency is also common and may influence the action and pharmacokinetics of antihypertensive drugs.
3. The elderly are much more likely to suffer coexisting diseases such as arthritis, chronic obstructive airways disease, Parkinsonism – all requiring drug therapy that may interact with their antihypertensive medication.

This chapter aims to consider the clinical pharmacology of antihypertensive drugs with particular reference to elderly patients. The drugs are considered by major therapeutic groups, with the clinically most important aspects of individual agents highlighted.

THIAZIDE DIURETICS

Thiazides have been extensively evaluated in major clinical trials and found to be effective both in respect of blood pressure reduction and reduction in morbidity and mortality in elderly hypertensives. At the time of writing no other drug group has been shown to be more effective in reducing the risks of stroke or myocardial infarction in hypertensive patients.

Mode of action

Despite more than 30 years of clinical use, the mode of action of these drugs in respect of their blood pressure lowering effect remains uncertain. The early response (days) relates to natriuresis, reduced extracellular volume and fall in cardiac output. In the longer-term (months) the net haemodynamic effect is a reduction in peripheral vascular resistance. Vascular reactivity to pressor agents is blunted, but the underlying mechanism is incompletely understood.

Pharmacokinetics

Most thiazides are well-absorbed after oral administration and presystemic metabolism is negligible. Volume of distribution and plasma protein binding are high. Elimination is partly by metabolism and partly by renal excretion of unchanged drug – the proportion varying between individual drugs within the group. Plasma elimination half-lives vary from 3 hours (bendrofluazide) to 90 hours (chlorthalidone). No specific data are available in elderly patients.

Dose–response relationships

There is no clear evidence relating plasma concentration of thiazides to their clinical effects. Dose–response relationships may vary with different endpoints: sodium excretion, potassium loss, blood glucose, blood pressure reduction. It has recently been convincingly shown that the blood pressure lowering effect of bendrofluazide is indistinguishable at daily doses of 1.25, 2.5, 5 and 10 mg (Carlsen *et al.*, 1990). Only the highest dose caused significant elevations in blood glucose, urate, creatinine and cholesterol. Similar data have now been reported for hydrochlorothiazide (Burris *et al.*, 1990) and cyclopenthiazide (Johnston *et al.*, 1991). One difficulty that remains is that some of the studies which confirmed the efficacy of thiazides in reducing morbidity and mortality in hypertension used higher doses than are currently recommended. It is assumed, and seems probable, that the very low doses now in vogue provide equivalent protection against stroke and myocardial events, but this has not yet been proven, and may never be.

Indications

Thiazides are first-line drugs for most forms of hypertension, and undoubtedly so in elderly patients. They are useful adjuncts to other antihypertensives, with a generally additive effect. Another important indication for thiazides is cardiac failure, especially when this is mild and renal function is well preserved. For more severe degrees of heart failure loop diuretics are used. Thiazides such as bendrofluazide may be added to loop diuretics in severe refractory heart failure (Channer et al., 1994).

Thiazides may inhibit the renal tubular secretion of calcium by about half. This may be a useful attribute in the treatment of renal stone disease, especially in patients with idiopathic hypercalciuria. Thiazide diuretics reduce urine volumes in patients with both pituitary and nephrogenic diabetes insipidus.

Contraindications

There are few absolute contraindications to the use of thiazides in hypertension, particularly if minimally effective doses are used. Pre-existing hyponatraemia, hypokalaemia and hyperuricaemia are likely to be worsened by thiazides and in such circumstances they should be avoided. Maturity onset diabetes or impaired glucose tolerance is a relative contraindication to moderate/high dose thiazides. Thiazides are not effective when the glomerular filtration rate falls below 30 ml/hour.

Adverse reactions

Biochemical/metabolic

The most serious direct effect of thiazides is profound hyponatraemia. This may be fatal. Frail elderly females are at greatest risk (Arieff, 1986; Ashraf et al., 1981).

Hypokalaemia is relatively common in patients taking thiazide diuretics, particularly at higher doses. The Medical Research Council's (MRC) trial in mild hypertension used a relatively high daily dose of bendrofluazide (10 mg), which was associated with an increased incidence of ventricular ectopic beats and arrhythmias associated with hypokalaemia (MRC Working Party on Mild to Moderate Hypertension, 1983). Nevertheless, overall cardiovascular mortality was not adversely affected (MRC Working Party, 1985a). It has further been suggested that thiazide-induced hypokalaemia does not result in increased ventricular ectopic activity or cardiac arrhythmias (Papademetriou et al., 1988). More recently, in a large cohort study, it has been reported that primary ventricular fibrillation in hypertension is closely related to diuretic-induced hypokalaemia and furthermore that potassium-sparing therapy ameliorates this effect (Siscovick et al., 1994). Some uncertainty remains, therefore, over this issue. Thiazide dosage should be kept to a minimum, the higher risk elderly should be monitored for hypokalaemia and if this is discovered a potassium-sparing combination should be used. This is more difficult than it sounds. Serum potassium is notoriously influenced by sampling and storage difficulties and many general practitioners may find it inconvenient to monitor this accurately. Hospital clinics may find it easier to monitor potassium levels, and this may be one of the advantages of shared-care schemes.

In the EWPHE trial the combination of hydrochlorothiazide with triamterene was used as first-line therapy in the active group (Amery et al., 1985).

Hypokalaemia was infrequently seen. In the MRC Elderly trial hydrochloro-thiazide with amiloride was used in the active group. Hypokalaemia was also infrequent (MRC Working Party, 1992). Dietary potassium intake may be poor in the elderly. Potassium supplements are a relatively inefficient method of returning serum potassium levels to normal and carry their own risks. Potassium-sparing drugs are effective and convenient, although care is required, particularly in patients with impaired renal function.

Thiazides have long been implicated in the elevation of total cholesterol, LDL cholesterol and triglycerides – indeed a considerable industry has devel-oped in promoting alternatives to the alleged adverse metabolic consequences of thiazides. This reputation has largely arisen from studies of questionable design, limited size, short duration and high dosage. However, even in the MRC mild hypertension trial, bendrofluazide 10 mg daily, compared with placebo, caused virtually no change in serum cholesterol over a 3-year follow-up period (Greenberg *et al.*, 1984). An overview of data from several other major trials concluded that, in the long term, thiazide diuretics have no adverse effect on plasma lipids (Moser, 1989). Few dose–response studies have been reported, but those that are available conclusively demonstrate that low dose thiazides do not increase lipid levels (Carlsen *et al.*, 1990). The adverse reputation of thiazides on lipids is largely unjustified. In particular, there is no evidence that these drugs have adverse effects on coronary heart disease in hypertensive patients. At least two large trials in which thiazides featured as first-line therapy have shown a convincing reduction in cardiovascular mortality.

Hyperuricaemia is a relatively common consequence of diuretic therapy and occasionally acute gout may be precipitated. Elevation in plasma urea is often observed in patients on thiazides, but progressive renal failure rarely develops. Nephrotoxicity of other drugs, e.g. non-steroidal anti-inflammatory drugs (NSAIDs), may be enhanced. Other biochemical abnormalities observed in association with thiazide use include hypercalcaemia, metabolic alkalosis and hypomagnesaemia.

Secondary aldosteronism is a feature of long-term thiazide use. The sodium retention induced by the increased aldosterone level tends to offset the hypoten-sive effect of the diuretic. If the thiazide is suddenly discontinued, rebound oedema may be a problem for a few weeks. This is especially problematic in middle aged females.

The concept of insulin resistance has recently been implicated in the patho-genesis of hypertension – particularly when associated with obesity and maturity onset diabetes. It had been speculated that thiazides may adversely affect this metabolic phenomenon but it has now been shown that low dose thiazides have virtually no effect on plasma insulin levels.

Miscellaneous

A number of idiosyncratic reactions have been associated with thiazides – acute pancreatitis, skin rashes, thrombocytopenia, haemolytic anaemia, aplastic anaemia, cholestatic jaundice. These could be related to chemical similarities between thiazides and sulphonamides, but most of these associations have arisen from case reports and verification of cause and effect relationship is often not possible. All of these reactions are rare.

Impotence was an unexpected symptom associated with thiazides in the MRC mild hypertension trial (MRC Working Party on Mild to Moderate Hypertension, 1983). The incidence was surprisingly high (23%) but the mechanism remains entirely unknown. It is unclear if lower doses cause this problem, which in any case is less likely to be a major consideration in an elderly as opposed to a younger population.

Drug interactions

Beneficial

Thiazides have a useful additive effect with most other antihypertensive drugs. The effects of angiotensin-converting enzyme inhibitors (ACE inhibitors) may be especially enhanced.

Adverse

Concomitant thiazide use may enhance the effects of initial doses of ACE inhibitors to such an extent that symptomatic hypotension may ensue (Webster *et al.*, 1987). It is advisable to discontinue diuretics at least on the day that an ACE inhibitor is started. Elderly patients may be more susceptible to any resultant hypotensive response.

Moderate to high doses of thiazide antagonize the action of sulphonylureas and may impair control in diabetic patients treated with these drugs.

Beta-adrenoceptor agonists such as salbutamol and terbutaline may cause hypokalaemia, especially if given parenterally in high doses, for example in patients with asthma. This effect may result in dangerously low potassium levels in patients requiring concurrent diuretic therapy. Corticosteroids may further exacerbate this problem.

Thiazide-related hypokalaemia may enhance the cardiotoxicity of digoxin. Intracellular potassium depletion may occur in the presence of a normal serum potassium.

Thiazides may antagonise the actions of uricosuric drugs by enhancing urate retention by the nephron. The effects of allopurinol and probenecid may be adversely affected in this way.

Thiazides inhibit the renal tubular excretion of lithium, with resultant high plasma levels and increased toxicity. The therapeutic 'window' for lithium is relatively narrow and this interaction carries a real risk of clinically important toxicity.

NSAIDs interact in two important ways with thiazides. First, thiazides may aggravate the nephrotoxicity of NSAID, especially in elderly patients with impaired renal function. These are not all equally potent, but azapropazone features consistently highly in surveys of relative toxicity (Langman *et al.*, 1994). NSAIDs in turn may antagonise the antihypertensive effect of thiazides. It is not clear if the underlying mechanism is non-specific – perhaps as a result of sodium retention – or if it may relate to inhibition of prostaglandin synthesis that could in turn reflect a mechanism of action of thiazides.

Individual characteristics

The most widely prescribed thiazides are bendrofluazide, cyclopenthiazide and hydrochlorothiazide. These have been extensively evaluated in large-scale clinical trials, and this has strengthened the case for choosing one of these as first-line antihypertensive therapy in routine practice. Although the information has come late, good dose–response data has now become available on how to judge the value of low-dose regimens of these drugs. Other frequently used thiazides are chlorthalidone, chlorothiazide and hydroflumethiazide.

Thiazides with particularly long half-lives, such as chlorthalidone and polythiazide, need to be used very cautiously in the elderly because of possible accumulation and biochemical disturbances. Some proprietary combinations, for example with beta-blockers and ACE inhibitors, contain doses of thiazide that are frequently excessive for an elderly population.

Major outcome trials in hypertension

All of the major outcome trials in hypertension to date have included thiazide diuretics either as first-line, alternative or add-on therapy in the active treatment group. No other group of antihypertensives has yet been shown to be superior in respect of prevention of stroke, myocardial infarction or overall mortality. The trials that have shown particularly the benefits of treating hypertension in elderly patients are: Coope and Warrender (1986), EWPHE (Amery *et al.*, 1985), SHEP (Systolic Hypertension in the Elderly Program (SHEP) Cooperative Research Group, 1991), MRC Elderly trial (MRC Working Party, 1992) and STOP-Hypertension (Dahlof *et al.*, 1991).

In summary, thiazides (often combined with potassium-sparing agents) have proved effective and well tolerated. They are at least as effective as any of the other major drug groups in respect of the reduction in blood pressure, and may be marginally more effective in respect of systolic blood pressure. Outcome data vary a little from study to study, but highly favourable results have been demonstrated in respect of virtually all of the cardiovascular complications of hypertension. These drugs can be recommended as a clear first choice in the elderly hypertensive.

LOOP DIURETICS

The most commonly used drugs in this group are frusemide and bumetanide. In elderly hypertensives they are reserved for patients with impaired renal function or co-existing cardiac failure.

Mode of action

In uncomplicated hypertension, loop diuretics are inferior to thiazides (Anderson *et al.*, 1971). The mode of action is probably similar to that of the thiazides, though this is incompletely understood. Reduction in peripheral resistance may occur during long-term therapy but loop diuretics may have a more prominent role through a fall in plasma volume. Unlike thiazides, loop diuretics retain their efficacy when glomerular filtration rate falls below 30% of normal and may thus be preferable in renal impairment. The powerful natriuretic effect of loop diuretics may also be useful when there is symptomatic heart failure. Loop diuretics may also be preferable when secondary fluid retention occurs, for example in refractory hypertension or during the concomitant administration of powerful vasodilator drugs such as minoxidil.

Pharmacokinetics

Both frusemide (65%) and bumetanide (80%) are well absorbed when given by mouth. Bioavailability is reduced by food. Both are partly cleared by glomerular filtration, partly by non-hepatic glucuronidation. Clearance is reduced in heart failure. Plasma elimination half-life is normally about 60 minutes.

Dose–response relationships

Unlike the thiazide diuretics, the natriuretic dose–response of loop diuretics is relatively steep. The dose–response with regard to blood pressure is much less well documented.

Indications

Loop diuretics are indicated in hypertension if there is co-existing renal insufficiency or cardiac failure, if the patient has refractory hypertension in spite of therapy with thiazides, beta-blockers, arteriolar dilators and ACE inhibitors. There is no place for these drugs in mild uncomplicated hypertension.

Contraindications

Loop diuretics must be used cautiously in renal impairment as the resultant volume depletion may further impair renal function. Known allergy to frusemide or sulphonamides contraindicates their subsequent use. Bumetanide may exhibit cross-sensitivity but the risks may be less frequent. Reliable data on this are understandably sparse.

Loop diuretics must be used with the greatest caution in patients with chronic liver disease because of the risks of electrolyte disturbance, hepatic decompensation and encephalopathy. Elderly patients are often very susceptible to acute volume depletion and minimally effective doses must be used.

Adverse reactions

Massive diuresis may occur with severe extracellular volume loss, hypotension and shock. A less severe degree of volume loss may lead to orthostatic hypotension. The elderly are particularly susceptible to these effects.

Biochemical disturbances are common – hyponatraemia, hypokalaemia, hypomagnesaemia, hyperuricaemia, elevated urea and creatinine. Hypergly-caemia may occur but is relatively uncommon. Depletion of potassium and magnesium is particularly likely in elderly patients with poor dietary intake. Increases in serum amylase may occur and, rarely, clinical pancreatitis.

High doses of loop diuretics may cause ototoxicity, particularly in patients with impaired renal function. Other uncommon adverse effects include skin rashes, thrombocytopenia and bone marrow depression.

In elderly patients, the rapid diuresis caused by loop diuretics may cause urinary difficulties, particularly in men with bladder outflow obstruction (retention) and in women with detrusor instability (incontinence). Patients travelling to attend hypertension clinics often avoid their morning dose of loop diuretic because of the inconvenience of urinary symptoms while on public transport!

Drug interactions

Beneficial

Generally loop diuretics enhance the effects of other antihypertensives. When ACE inhibitors are added to patients on diuretics, severe hypotension may result, especially in elderly patients with heart failure. The combination of loop diuretic with thiazide is an especially useful combination in refractory heart failure, though its very potency may cause problems with electrolyte homeostasis (Channer *et al.*, 1994).

b) Adverse

Diuretic-induced hypokalaemia increases the cardiotoxicity of digoxin. The hypokalaemia may be enhanced by the co-administration of corticosteroids and/or beta-sympathomimetics. Loop diuretics may enhance the ototoxicity of aminoglycosides and the nephrotoxicity of first generation cephalosporins. Serious lithium toxicity may occur when loop diuretics are co-administered.

NSAIDs partly antagonise the diuretic and antihypertensive effect of diuretics. Nephrotoxicity also is enhanced during co-administration.

Major outcome trials in hypertension

None have been reported.

POTASSIUM-SPARING DIURETICS

The two most frequently used drugs in this category are amiloride and tri-amterene. Spironolactone is used in primary aldosteronism.

Mode of action

Both amiloride and triamterene act directly on the distal tubule to cause a fall in electrical potential across the epithelium. A mild natriuresis is induced and excretion of potassium and magnesium is not altered. This effect is independent of the action of aldosterone. Both drugs are most frequently used in combination with a thiazide or loop diuretic. In this situation they inhibit potassium excretion. This is a much more efficient method of maintaining serum potassium levels than the addition of potassium supplements.

Spironolactone is a competitive antagonist of aldosterone at the distal tubule. Its main role in the management of hypertension is in the medical treatment of primary aldosteronism.

Pharmacokinetics

Amiloride is incompletely absorbed, widely distributed, and excreted unchanged in the urine, with a plasma elimination half-life of approximately 8 hours.

Triamterene also shows considerable interindividual variation in absorption and presystemic metabolism. Less than 10% of the urinary excretion of tri-amterene is as the unchanged drug. Elimination half-life is approximately 2 hours.

Spironolactone is very lipophilic, with variable absorption that is enhanced by food. It is very extensively metabolised to multiple metabolites, many of which have biological activity. The principal active metabolite is canrenone. Plasma elimination half-life of the parent drug is about 1 hour.

Dose–response relationships

Amiloride

This has not been clearly established in hypertension, though the recommended dose range is narrow, from 5–20 mg daily. As commonly prescribed, in combination with a thiazide diuretic, the usual ratio is 5 mg amiloride to 25 mg hydrochlorothiazide.

Triamterene

Triamterene is not used alone in hypertension. As most commonly used, in combination with a thiazide diuretic, the usual ratio is 50 mg triamterene to 25 mg hydrochlorothiazide.

Spironolactone

In essential hypertension the dose–response relationship with respect to blood pressure is flat, and there is little advantage in using more than 100 mg/day. In primary aldosteronism, correction of the hypokalaemic alkalosis can often be achieved by a similar modest dose, although control of the blood pressure on monotherapy may require titration of up to 400 mg daily.

Indications

In hypertension, amiloride and triamterene are almost exclusively used in combination with a thiazide diuretic. A number of large-scale trials attest to their efficacy in elderly hypertensives when used in this way. Apart from hypertension, amiloride and triamterene are also used in combination with thiazides or loop diuretics in the treatment of heart failure and ascites due to chronic liver disease. They may also be used in the management of primary aldosteronism, especially when spironolactone is poorly tolerated.

Spironolactone is indicated for primary aldosteronism and in the treatment of refractory oedema due to heart failure, cirrhosis, nephrotic syndrome or malignant ascites. It is no longer recommended in essential hypertension.

Contraindications

Dangerous hyperkalaemia may be induced or exaggerated with all of these drugs. This is especially likely in patients with renal insufficiency. Amiloride should not be used in diabetes.

Drug interactions

Beneficial

The combination of amiloride or triamterene with a thiazide diuretic results in a highly effective, well-tolerated and extensively tested antihypertensive formulation.

Adverse

All potassium-sparing drugs may cause dangerous hyperkalaemia if potassium supplements are added or if they are combined with each other. Hyperkalaemia may also result from the combination of potassium-sparing drugs with ACE inhibitors.

Potassium-sparing drugs are usually prescribed in combination with thiazide or loop diuretics to prevent or correct hypokalaemia. Occasionally an enhanced natriuretic response occurs with such combination therapy, with resultant hyponatraemia. This is most frequently seen when these drugs are used in proprietary fixed dose combinations with hydrochlorothiazide. These may contain unnecessarily high dosages of the individual constituents. Especially in the elderly patient, the minimal effective dose should always be used for hypertension.

Amiloride and triamterene may reduce the renal clearance of lithium, with resultant toxicity.

Amiloride does not impair glucose tolerance but some diabetic patients may be susceptible to hyperkalaemia and it is best avoided in such patients.

Amiloride is frequently prescribed with digoxin in order to prevent thiazide- or loop diuretic-induced hypokalaemia, but reduced renal clearance of digoxin may result and close monitoring to avoid digoxin toxicity is recommended. Spironolactone has a similar effect.

Major outcome studies in hypertension

Amiloride was combined with hydrochlorothiazide in the diuretic regimen of the MRC Elderly Trial (MRC Working Party, 1992), and in the STOP-Hypertension trial (Dahlof *et al.*, 1991).

Triamterene was combined with hydrochlorothiazide in the EWPHE trial (Amery *et al.*, 1985).

In the Puget Sound cohort study, the addition of either triamterene or spirono-lactone to hydrochlorothiazide or chlorthalidone was associated with a reduced risk of primary cardiac arrest in hypertensive patients (Siscovick *et al.*, 1994).

CENTRALLY ACTING DRUGS

Although no longer regarded as first-line agents, centrally acting antihyper-tensive drugs remain very useful as second- or third-line therapy or when contraindications to first-line drugs are present. Methyldopa is still widely prescribed. Clonidine is seldom used now in the UK, while rilmenidine and moxonidine are too recent to have found their place in therapy.

Mode of action

Both methyldopa and clonidine are now thought to act primarily as central alpha$_2$-agonists, resulting in a reduction in efferent sympathetic tone. By contrast, the effects of rilmenidine and moxonidine are mediated primarily by stimulation of imidazoline I$_2$ receptors in the rostral ventrolateral medulla.

Pharmacokinetics

Methyldopa is characterised by incomplete absorption and extensive 'first-pass' metabolism that is heavily influenced by food. This makes dosing rather unpre-dictable, with a bioavailability of 25%. Metabolism in the liver to sulphated con-jugates is the principal route, whereas metabolism in noradrenergic neurones to alpha-methylnoradrenaline is responsible for the antihypertensive action of the drug. Plasma elimination half-life is less than 2 hours, although the clinical effects last considerably longer than this.

Clonidine, by contrast, is almost completely absorbed, with very little pre-systemic metabolism. About 60% is excreted unchanged by the kidney, the remainder by hepatic microsomal oxidation. Elimination half-life from plasma is 24 hours.

Dose–response relationships

Methyldopa

Daily doses of up to 4.5 g have been used, but, as with many other antihyper-tensive drugs, lower doses may be just as effective while minimising side effects.

There is no clear relationship between dose and antihypertensive effect. The usual starting dose is 250 mg twice daily, and even half that may be appropriate in older patients.

Clonidine

The magnitude of the blood pressure lowering effect and the frequency of central side effects of clonidine increase with increasing plasma concentrations. At very high doses the blood pressure lowering effect declines as a result of post-sympathetic alpha$_1$ agonist action on resistance arterioles.

Indications

In uncomplicated hypertension in the elderly, methyldopa is recommended 'add-on' therapy in the event of contraindications, intolerance or resistance to first-line drugs. The drug is particularly useful as it has no major adverse effects on cardiac, renal or respiratory function. Contrary to popular myth, methyldopa is a well-tolerated second-line drug in elderly hypertensives (Amery *et al.*, 1985).

Clonidine is now seldom used because of its adverse effect profile. It compares unfavourably with other drugs used as monotherapy in middle-aged men (Materson *et al.*, 1993). No large-scale safety or efficacy data are available in elderly hypertensives.

Contraindications

Methyldopa must be avoided in patients with previous hypersensitivity to the drug, known postural hypotension, liver disease or depressive illness.

Clonidine should be avoided in patients with bradycardia or cardiac conduction defects.

Adverse reactions

Methyldopa

Hypersensitivity reactions are the most unpredictable and dangerous. Though relatively rare, fatalities have been documented as a result of hepatitis (Toghill *et al.*, 1974), myocarditis (Mullick and McAllister, 1977), and haemolytic anaemia (Worlledge *et al.*, 1966). Less serious abnormalities such as abnormal liver function tests or positive Coomb's tests, drug fever and pancreatitis occur in up to 20% of patients. Central side effects are also relatively frequent and may necessitate withdrawal of therapy in about 20% of patients, particularly at higher doses (Croog *et al.*, 1986). These effects include sedation, sleep disturbance, dry mouth, nasal stuffiness, psychotic reactions and depression. Parkinsonism may be induced or aggravated. A rebound syndrome has been described. Adverse effects related directly to its blood pressure lowering effect include postural hypotension. This is particularly important in elderly patients prone to postural instability.

Clonidine

The most feared complication of clonidine therapy for hypertension is a with-drawal syndrome after the drug is deliberately or inadvertently discontinued (Weber, 1980). Within a three-day period blood pressure may rise rapidly, and even overshoot, and patients may develop symptoms of tremor, tachycardia, headache, vasomotor instability, insomnia, psychiatric disturbance, nausea and vomiting. The clinical features may resemble a phaeochromocytoma crisis, and opiate or alcohol withdrawal. Plasma concentrations of noradrenaline are increased (Reid *et al.*, 1977). The problem may be particularly severe in patients with preceding severe hypertension. Fatalities have been recorded (Webster *et al.*, 1974). The rise in blood pressure may be at least partly related to the effects of noradrenaline on peripheral alpha receptors – these may be exaggerated by co-administration of non-selective beta-blockers. It is largely because of this syndrome that clonidine is now seldom used in the UK.

Other central side effects are also problematic. Sedation and dry mouth are very common and constipation, sleep disturbance and postural hypotension may be especially troublesome in older patients.

Bradycardia and impaired atrioventricular conduction may result from the reduction in cardiac sympathetic drive, and are especially problematic in patients with underlying cardiac disease.

Although the drug is a very effective antihypertensive, comparative studies have shown it to be less well tolerated than most of the conventional alternatives (Materson *et al.*, 1993).

Drug interactions

Beneficial

Both methyldopa and clonidine combine satisfactorily with thiazide diuretics.

Adverse

Occasionally, the use of methyldopa in combination therapy with other anti-hypertensives results in excessive hypotension (Webster *et al.*, 1977). Hypotensive reactions have also been described when methyldopa is combined with levodopa, phenothiazines or general anaesthetics.

Methyldopa may enhance the pressor effects of sympathomometics. The central effects of clonidine, especially drowsiness, will be augmented by other centrally acting drugs such as alcohol, antihistamines, barbiturates, benzodiazepines, phenothiazines, etc. Non-selective beta-blockers may exacerbate the rebound hypertension that occurs after clonidine withdrawal.

Major outcome trials

Methyldopa

In the EWPHE trial (Amery *et al.*, 1985), 145/416 (35%) patients in the active treatment group were treated with methyldopa in doses up to 2 g/day used to supplement first line treatment with 'Dyazide' (hydrochlorothiazide + triamterene).

Cardiac mortality was significantly reduced by 38%. Cardiovascular morbidity and stroke mortality were also reduced. Patients tolerated the drug well.

In a well-documented quality of life study, 20% of the methyldopa treated group withdrew from active treatment because of adverse effects (Croog *et al.*, 1986). However, this study used a relatively large dosage regimen.

Clonidine

Clonidine was used as monotherapy in two large parallel group comparisons (Materson *et al.*, 1993; Treatment of Mild Hypertension Research Group, 1991). Overall, clonidine matched all of the other first line agents in respect of efficacy in lowering blood pressure but was least well tolerated. No large-scale morbidity/mortality study has been reported using clonidine as first-line therapy.

BETA-BLOCKERS

This large group of drugs remains, with thiazides, the mainstay of drug therapy for hypertension as established in major outcome studies. All of these drugs have similar effects on blood pressure. Individual characteristics of drugs in this group are summarised in Table 5.1. Occasionally their ancillary properties may be clinically useful in selected patients, but there is considerable logic in preferring a low dose of a highly selective agent that can be given once a day.

Mode of action

The mechanism by which beta-blockers reduce blood pressure remains unclear. Competitive blockade of $beta_1$-adrenoceptors seems fundamental and $beta_2$-blockade contributes little to the effect (Robb *et al.*, 1988). Ancillary properties such as alpha antagonism or direct vasodilator activity may enhance the blood pressure lowering effect but may also contribute to postural or first dose hypotension (Webster *et al.*, 1985). Various mechanisms have been suggested, including central inhibition of sympathetic tone, presynaptic inhibition of sympathetic nerve transmission, inhibition of baroreflex sensitivity, inhibition of renin secretion and direct effect on vasomotor tone (Cruickshank *et al.*, 1988). It is possible that several of these apply and that the predominant mechanism may vary between individuals. For example, in patients with a 'hyperdynamic' circulation, the suppression of heart rate and cardiac output may be important. On the other hand, in some patients with renovascular hypertension, the inhibition of renin release may result in dramatic falls in blood pressure.

Pharmacokinetics

In general, lipid-soluble beta-blockers, such as propranolol, are characterised by complete absorption, large volume of distribution and extensive hepatic metabolism, whereas water-soluble beta-blockers, such as atenolol, are less

Table 5.1 Principal characteristics of beta-blockers

	Pharmacodynamics			Drug	Pharmacokinetics			
Beta$_1$-selectivity	ISA*	Solubility	Extra		Absorption	Metabolism	$t_{1/2}$ (h)†	1st pass (%)
Yes	No	Water		Atenolol	60	No	10	0
Yes	No	Lipid		Metoprolol	95	Yes	4	50
Yes	Yes	Water		Practolol	90	No	13	0
Yes	Yes	Water	Vasodilator	Celiprolol	20	No	70	0
Yes	Yes	Lipid		Bisoprolol	95	Yes	12	70
No	No	Lipid		Propranolol	90	Yes	4	70
No	No	Water		Nadolol	30	No	24	0
No	No	Water	Class III antiarrhythmic	Sotalol	90	No	15	0
No	No	Water		Timolol	90	Yes	5	60
No	No	Lipid	Alpha-antagonist	Labetolol	90	Yes	6	70
No	No	Lipid		Oxprenolol	90	Yes	2	80
No	No	Lipid		Alprenolol	90	Yes	3	90
No	No	Lipid		Penbutolol	90	Yes	26	70
No	No	Water		Pindolol	90	Yes	5	20
Yes	Yes	Lipid		Acebutolol	70	Yes	7	30

*ISA = intrinsic sympathomimetic activity; †$t_{1/2}$ = elimination half-life well absorbed, less extensively distributed and are excreted unchanged by the kidney. The pharmacokinetic properties of the more widely used beta-blockers are also summarised in Table 5.1.

Propranolol is the prototype drug of this group. It is characterised by rapid absorption and extensive, variable, flow-dependent 'first-pass' metabolism. As with other lipid-soluble drugs, this property necessitates careful dose-titration to ensure optimal response. It is highly bound to albumin and alpha$_1$-acid glycoprotein and distributed to extravascular tissues, including the brain. Plasma elimination half-life after long-term therapy is up to 6 hours. In the elderly, clearance of propranolol is reduced by about 50%, with resultant plasma concentrations that are 3–4 times higher than in younger patients. Sustained-release preparations are available that slow the absorption and increase the elimination half-life to 12 hours. Elimination may also be longer in obesity, hypothyroidism and in patients with chronic liver disease, and shorter in thyrotoxicosis.

Atenolol is the market leader. It is hydrophilic, incompletely absorbed and not subject to hepatic metabolism. As a result, interindividual variability in drug levels is less than for most other beta-blockers, and not greatly affected by other drugs. Atenolol is not widely distributed, and in particular, reaches much lower concentrations in the brain than lipophilic beta-blockers, with fewer central side effects. Elimination is principally by renal excretion, which is reduced in the elderly in direct proportion to the decline in renal function.

As a general rule, therefore, beta-blockers can be expected to exhibit higher plasma concentrations for a given dose in the elderly compared with younger patients, whether the drug is cleared by hepatic or renal mechanisms, and dosages should be tailored accordingly. Antihypertensive efficacy may not increase with increasing plasma concentrations, but adverse effects may.

Dose–response relationships

Suppression of exercise heart rate exhibits a log–linear relationship with the plasma concentration of beta-blockers (Harron *et al.*, 1981). By contrast, plasma levels bear little relationship to changes in blood pressure. In hypertension, the dose–response relationship between beta-blockers and hypotensive effect is relatively flat (Jeffers *et al.*, 1977). During the early development of these drugs, daily doses of up to 4 g propranolol and 600 mg atenolol were used, whereas it is now recognised that only a fraction of these doses is required for optimal effect. It is now widely accepted that in mild to moderate essential hypertension, most major groups of antihypertensives are of similar blood pressure-lowering efficacy, and that within the beta-blocker group, the individual agents are equally effective (Davidson *et al.*, 1976).

Indications

In hypertension, beta-blockers may be rather more effective in patients with normal or high renin levels. Such profiling is not a realistic proposition in routine practice. Elderly patients tend to have low renin hypertension and beta-blockers may be expected to be rather less effective in this group. This hypothesis is supported by comparative studies showing rather poorer responses in elderly Black males (Materson *et al.*, 1993). The MRC elderly trial showed that a thiazide-based regimen might have advantages over an atenolol-based regimen in elderly hypertensives (MRC Working Party, 1992).

Concurrent illness such as angina, paroxysmal supraventricular tachycardia, previous myocardial infarction, migraine and thyrotoxicosis each provide additional reasons to choose a beta-blocker.

Non-smokers benefit more from beta-blockers than smokers (Medical Research Council Working Party, 1985b). Men may benefit more than women and Whites more than Blacks, though in accelerated hypertension both propranolol (Buhler *et al.*, 1973) and atenolol (Isles *et al.*, 1986) are highly effective, irrespective of race. In a more acute context, beta-blockers are particularly indicated in patients with aortic dissection. This is often associated with rather severe hypertension. 'Conservative' medical management of such patients (often elderly) should involve aggressive reduction of blood pressure to the lowest level tolerated by the patient. The particular haemodynamic advantage of beta-blockade in this situation is the reduction in the rate of rise in aortic pressure during systole and resultant reduction in wall stress.

Other indications for the use of beta-blockers are summarised in Table 5.2.

Table 5.2   Indications for beta-blockers

Cardiac
   angina pectoris
   aortic dissection
   arrhythmias
   hypertension
   myocardial infarction

Non-cardiac
   anxiety
   glaucoma
   migraine
   thyrotoxicosis

Contraindications

Beta-blockers are absolutely contraindicated in asthma. They should be used with the greatest care in patients with heart failure, cardiac conduction disturbances, severe peripheral vascular disease, Raynaud's phenomenon, and diabetes mellitus.

Adverse reactions

Airways obstruction is the most serious adverse effect of beta-blockers. Fatalities have occurred, even after the administration of timolol in the form of eye drops (Committee on Safety of Medicines, 1981; Fraunfelder and Barker,

1984). This route bypasses the presystemic hepatic microsomal enzyme system and results in significant systemic effects in susceptible patients. Even selective drugs are not free from this problem and a history of asthma is an absolute contraindication to the use of these drugs.

Beta-blockers may also precipitate heart failure, especially in patients suboptimally treated with diuretics and ACE inhibitors. Frank heart failure may be unmasked in patients with previously unrecognised disease. These patients may be dependent on activation of their sympathetic drive to the heart to maintain their cardiac output and if this is blocked, myocardial function will decline.

Cardiac conduction disturbances may also be worsened by beta-blockade. This is especially important in older patients with sick sinus syndrome. Drugs with intrinsic sympathomimetic activity, e.g. pindolol or oxprenolol, may be preferable if it is thought important to avoid bradycardia.

Tired legs and cold extremities are the commonest side effects of beta-blockers, even in otherwise normal subjects (Cruickshank, 1981). Patients with Raynaud's phenomenon and severe peripheral vascular disease are especially vulnerable. Claudication may be worsened, though this is by no means inevitable, but skin circulation is almost always adversely affected.

Beta-blockers may be used in diabetes, but particular care must be taken in patients prone to hypoglycaemia, as the tachycardia may be masked and the recovery in blood glucose delayed (Davidson *et al.*, 1977; Deacon *et al.*, 1977). Non-selective drugs should be avoided.

Central side effects, such as depression, sleep disturbance, increased dreaming and nightmares are associated with the lipophilic beta-blockers, which pass readily across the blood–brain barrier.

Sudden withdrawal of beta-blockers may result in a withdrawal syndrome of tachycardia, tremor, headache and sweating. Angina may occur and may progress to myocardial infarction and death (Alderman *et al.*, 1974). The problem is particularly serious in patients with underlying coronary disease, but as this may be occult in asymptomatic hypertensives it is always preferable to discontinue these drugs slowly. The syndrome may relate to increased myocardial sensitivity to endogenous catecholamines, up-regulation of beta-receptors, or progression of underlying coronary disease. A rapid rise in exercise heart rate, coupled with instability of arterial plaques, may be of critical importance.

Drug interactions

Beneficial

Beta-blockers combine usefully with most other antihypertensives, with which their antihypertensive effect is generally additive. They are particularly useful in combination with vasodilator drugs such as dihydropyridines, hydralazine and minoxidil as they suppress the reflex tachycardia associated with these drugs that can cause unwanted symptoms.

Adverse

Beta-blockers augment the effects of cardioinhibitory drugs such as verapamil, diltiazem, lignocaine, disopyramide and flecainide. As a result patients may suffer heart failure, bradycardia, conduction defects and even asystole. The negative chronotropic effect and delayed atrio-ventricular conduction actions of digoxin may also be enhanced.

The bronchodilatory effects of beta-agonist drugs such as salbutamol and terbutaline are also antagonised. Not only may asthma be precipitated, but it may also become more refractory to conventional treatment in these circumstances.

Unopposed alpha-pressor reactions to catecholamines may occur if a beta-blocker is co-prescribed during insulin-induced hypoglycaemic reactions, clonidine withdrawal or phaeochromocytoma crises. These may be less likely with beta$_1$-selective blockers.

The co-administration of vasodilator drugs, such as the dihydropyridines, may exacerbate any tendency to rebound myocardial ischaemia when beta-blockers are suddenly withdrawn.

The antihypertensive effect of beta-blockers may be attenuated by non-steroidal anti-inflammatory drugs. It is not known if this is a prostaglandin-specific or non-specific effect.

Major outcome studies

Beta-blockers have been included in the active treatment regimens of a number of major trials in hypertension, including: MRC mild hypertension trial using propranolol (MRC Working Party, 1985b), Australian mild hypertension trial using timolol (Management Committee of the Australian National Blood Pressure Study, 1980), HAPPHY using metoprolol and atenolol (Wilhelmson *et al.*, 1987), IPPPSH with oxprenolol (IPPPSH Collaborative Group, 1985), MRC elderly trial with atenolol (MRC Working Party, 1992), SHEP using atenolol (Systolic Hypertension in the Elderly Program (SHEP) Cooperative Research Group, 1991), STOP-Hypertension using pindolol (Dahlof *et al.*, 1991) and TOHMS using atenolol (Treatment of Mild Hypertension Research Group, 1991).

In brief, the beta-blockers reduced blood pressure and were reasonably well tolerated. Elderly patients and smokers responded less well to beta-blockers than to thiazides. The incidence of strokes was reduced. Myocardial events were also reduced but by a relatively smaller amount. Elderly patients benefit more than younger patients because their absolute risk is greater. Contrary to expectations there is no evidence from these trials that beta-blockers are particularly 'cardio-protective' when used in hypertension. They are not demonstrably superior to diuretics and in some of the trials were inferior.

CALCIUM CHANNEL ANTAGONISTS

The calcium channel antagonists have been classified by the World Health Organisation into three main categories on the basis of their pharmacological profile and haemodynamic effects (Table 5.3). Each of the three categories may be used in the treatment of hypertension.

Table 5.3 Calcium antagonists

	Angina	Hypertension	Supraventricular tachycardia	Raynaud's	Hypertrophic obstructive cardiomyopathy	Post-myocardial infarction
Verapamil	+++	++	+++	0	++	0
Diltiazem	++	++	++	+	0	–
Dihydropyridines	+	++	0	++	0	0

Calcium antagonists – some characteristics of individual drugs

Amlodipine   slow onset, long half-life
Felodipine   vascular selective (?)
Isradipine
Lacidipine   long-acting
Nicardipine   vascular selective (?)
Nifedipine   prototype drug
Nimodipine   indicated in subarachnoid haemorrhage
Nisoldipine   vascular selectivity (?)
Nitrendipine

+++ = most useful; 0 = not useful; + = uncertain

Mode of action

All three categories act as selective dilators of arterioles in the systemic, pulmonary and coronary circulations. Blood pressure falls promptly after oral administration. The dihydropyridines are accompanied by a reflex tachycardia. This is much less marked after diltiazem, and verapamil tends to produce a slowing of heart rate. At high doses all of these drugs may exhibit a negative inotropic effect, although this is greatest with verapamil and diltiazem.

Pharmacokinetics

There are some important differences, even within the dihydropyridine group, that have implications for clinical practice. Nifedipine is the prototype dihydropyridine. It is very rapidly and completely absorbed, but undergoes extensive presystemic metabolism. The rapid absorption has been associated with the high incidence of vasodilator side effects such as headache, flushing and tachycardia. The 'first-pass' effect shows considerable interindividual variability and necessitates careful dose-titration. Plasma elimination half-life averages 4 hours. Various sustained release formulations have been developed to try to overcome some of these kinetic disadvantages.

By contrast amlodipine is more slowly absorbed, and is not subject to significant presystemic metabolism. Plasma elimination half-life averages 36 hours. This profile offers advantages in terms of patient compliance and may help minimise vasodilator side effects.

Both diltiazem and verapamil resemble nifedipine in their pharmacokinetic properties and sustained release formulations have been developed in an attempt to overcome these.

The clearance of these drugs tends to be reduced in the elderly, and the plasma elimination half-life prolonged, but this is seldom of major clinical significance.

Dose–response relationships

As with most other antihypertensive drugs, calcium channel antagonists have been introduced into routine clinical practice at unnecessarily high dosage. This is partly responsible for the high incidence of side effects associated with this group of drugs. For drugs exhibiting extensive presystemic metabolism, stepwise dose titration is recommended to find the minimum dosage that controls the blood pressure while minimising the adverse effects. For nifedipine the effective daily dose ranges from 10 mg to 80 mg. For amlodipine the range may be narrower – 2.5 to 10 mg daily – but failure to start at the lowest dose often results in similar difficulties. The effective daily dose range for diltiazem is 120–360 mg, and for verapamil 80–480 mg. The lowest possible starting dose should always be used.

Indications

In the elderly hypertensive, the calcium antagonists should all be regarded as second- or third-line drugs. They are particularly useful in hypertensive patients with airway obstruction, peripheral vascular disease, renal impairment or diabetes, when other drugs are contraindicated. They have additional attributes that may be useful in hypertensive patients with co-existing disease. In angina, verapamil and diltiazem may be preferred because they tend not to increase heart rate and may be more effective in the control of symptoms than dihydropyridines. Both may also be useful in patients with supraventricular tachycardias.

Dihydropyridines have an ancillary use in the symptomatic treatment of Raynaud's phenomenon.

Nifedipine improves cardiac performance and delays the need for valve replacement in patients with aortic regurgitation (Scognamiglio *et al.*, 1994). This diagnosis should always be considered in patients with isolated systolic hypertension or with a particularly wide pulse pressure.

Contraindications

All calcium channel antagonists must be used with great caution in patients with heart failure. At higher doses nifedipine may exhibit a negative inotropic effect. It is probable that amlodipine, felodipine, isradipine, lacidipine and nicardipine are relatively more selective for arterioles than the myocardium and it is not certain that these drugs would make heart failure worse. Diltiazem and verapamil are much more likely to exhibit negative inotropic effects and they should not be used in patients with impaired left ventricular function. This is a very important limitation on their use in elderly populations.

Diltiazem and verapamil both suppress atrioventricular conduction and should be avoided in patients with sick sinus syndrome or with second or third degree heart block.

Calcium antagonists are also best avoided in patients with aortic stenosis as a rapid reduction in peripheral resistance may lead to severe hypotension and syncope in such patients. By a similar mechanism, nifedipine has been reported to cause sudden cardiovascular collapse in patients with pulmonary hypertension (Anon, 1991).

Adverse reactions

Vasodilator side effects are very commonly associated with dihydropyridines. Some of the effects clearly relate to rapid absorption of the active drug and to both its direct action on vessels and the reflex tachycardia that results. Such effects include facial flushing, headache, tachycardia, palpitations, chest pain and conjunctival irritation. With more prolonged administration, leg oedema becomes more pronounced, especially in women, and frequently necessitates discontinuation of therapy. This is not caused by heart failure or by 'fluid retention' but by local vascular effects, including relaxation of precapillary arterioles. In hypertension, approximately 30% of patients will experience adverse symptoms on dihydropyridines and at least 10% will discontinue therapy as a result (Benson and Webster, 1995).

Vasodilator side effects are less troublesome with diltiazem and verapamil, but constipation can be rather troublesome with the latter drug.

Heart failure may result from the negative inotropic action of calcium channel antagonists. Clinical trial results have shown that in patients with impaired left ventricular function after myocardial infarction, diltiazem *increases* mortality (Goldstein *et al.*, 1991; Multicentre Dilthiazem Postinfarction Research Group, 1988). Unfortunately this information does not appear to be widely appreciated and many patients continue to be put at risk by the imprudent use of this drug for post-infarction angina. Neither verapamil nor dihydropyridines have been shown to have such a deleterious effect. However, as a general rule these drugs should *not* be prescribed routinely in the post-infarct patient as they have not been shown to be useful in reducing mortality or reinfarction. Until further evidence is forthcoming from clinical trials they should all be avoided in patients with overt heart failure.

Cardiac conduction disturbances are frequently associated with diltiazem and verapamil, and great care should be taken in the use of these drugs in patients with pre-existing cardiac conduction disorders.

Other effects attributed to calcium channel antagonists include gingival hyperplasia, worsening angina, rashes and joint pains.

Drug interactions

Beneficial

Calcium channel antagonists have generally additive effects with other antihypertensive and antianginal drugs. Some of their ancillary actions are complementary, for example the combination of dihydropyridine with a beta-blocker enhances the desired effect while minimising side effects.

Adverse

The risk of cardiac conduction disturbances is greatly enhanced when either diltiazem or verapamil is combined with beta-blockers. Heart failure is also more likely. Verapamil should not be given intravenously to patients already receiving beta-blocker or digoxin as complete heart block and even asystole may result.

Both diltiazem and verapamil increase plasma concentrations of digoxin, theophylline, lithium and cyclosporin.

Major outcome trials

Diltiazem

In patients who have experienced myocardial infarction, diltiazem offers no benefit in terms of reinfarction or mortality, and it increases mortality in patients with impaired ventricular function (Goldstein *et al.*, 1991). It is an effective antianginal drug but has not been shown to have a useful role in primary prevention of myocardial infarction. It is an effective antihypertensive drug, though it may need to be titrated to high doses to obtain the full effect (Materson *et al.*, 1993). Limited data are available from major outcome studies. Diltiazem is being evaluated as 'add-on' therapy to bendrofluazide or lisinopril in hypertensive patients over the age of 80 in the HYVET trial (Bulpitt *et al.*, 1994).

Verapamil

Antianginal and antihypertensive efficacy is not in doubt. No major advantages have been demonstrated for verapamil over other antianginal or antihypertensive drugs in respect of morbidity or mortality.

Dihydropyridines

Despite much promotional activity by the pharmaceutical industry and some academic centres, there is no evidence that these drugs are superior to other groups in respect of morbidity and mortality, either in relation to angina or hypertension. It is important to bear these major primary endpoints in mind when evaluating efficacy. In one well-publicised study, nifedipine was claimed to retard the angiographic progression of coronary artery disease (Hugenholz *et al.*, 1990). However, there was a substantial excess of deaths in the nifedipine treated group. Nifedipine has been evaluated in patients after myocardial infarction, with little evidence either of a clinically important benefit or added risk (Israeli Sprint Study Group, 1988; Wilcox *et al.*, 1986). Preliminary data from the Shanghai Trial of Nifedipine in the Elderly (STONE) suggests a reduction in study terminating events (see Appendix for further details). Dihydropyridines (nitrendipine) are being evaluated as first-line antihypertensive therapy in the elderly in the SYST-EUR (Amery *et al.*, 1991) and SYST-CHINA (Systolic Hypertension in the Elderly's Collaborative Group Co-ordinating Center, 1992) trials currently in progress, though the results are unlikely to be available until the end of the century.

In a recent series of publications, serious concerns have been raised about the safety of calcium antagonists with regard to post-myocardial infarction and hypertension. In a meta-analysis of post-infarction studies it was suggested that the use of nifedipine in moderate to high doses caused an increase in total mortality (Furberg *et al.*, 1995). A significant dose–response relationship with increased mortality heightened the plausibility of the results. In a separate population-based, case-controlled study in hypertensive patients, the use of short-acting calcium antagonists, especially in high doses, was associated with an increased risk of myocardial infarction (Psaty *et al.*, 1995). Compared with diuretics and beta-blockers, calcium antagonist use was associated with an approximate 60% increased risk of myocardial infarction. These reports have generated heated debate (Horton, 1995; Kloner, 1995; Opie and Messerli, 1995; Yusuf, 1995). Despite the undoubted limitations of these studies (Buring *et al.*, 1995), at the very least they have generated the hypothesis that some calcium antagonists may have adverse effects on morbidity and mortality. That hypothesis now needs to be tested in prospective randomised trials in the same way that diuretics and beta-blockers have been tested. Until the issue is clarified, a degree of caution in prescribing these drugs would seem appropriate.

ANGIOTENSIN CONVERTING ENZYME INHIBITORS

A large number of drugs in this group are now widely available, and a huge world literature surrounds their use. Initially introduced for patients with refractory and/or renovascular hypertension, they are now used in all grades of hypertension. In recent years they have also established a central role in the management of heart failure and myocardial infarction, where extensive and convincing evidence is now available to show that ACE inhibitors reduce morbidity and mortality. Unfortunately data of similar quality are currently lacking in respect of primary prevention in hypertension.

Mode of action

All drugs in this group act as competitive inhibitors of angiotensin-converting enzyme. This enzyme mediates both the conversion of angiotensin I to angiotensin II and the catabolism of bradykinin. All ACE inhibitors reduce peripheral resistance, and hence lower blood pressure. Inhibition of the converting enzyme results in greatly reduced concentrations of the circulating pressor hormone angiotensin II, and a resultant reduction in aldosterone secretion (Atkinson et al., 1982). ACE inhibitors would thus be expected to be particularly effective in high renin conditions such as renovascular hypertension. To a certain extent this is the case, though it is now appreciated that ACE inhibitors will reduce blood pressure even in patients with normal or low plasma renin levels. Originally, it was thought that the principal site of action of these drugs was in the lung. As experience has accumulated with these drugs it has become apparent that converting enzyme is present in endothelial, epithelial and neuronal cells at numerous other sites, such as the adrenal, brain, gut, kidney and placenta, and these may also be important in some patients (Morgan, 1993). It has been claimed that some ACE inhibitors are more 'vascular selective' than others, and that this may have implications for vascular remodelling, but this has yet to be proven in clinical practice.

Pharmacokinetics

The pharmacokinetics of the ACE inhibitors are summarised in Table 5.4. Captopril is the prototype drug of the group. It is well-absorbed with a peak plasma concentration seen within 1 hour of oral dosing. A small amount of hepatic conjugation occurs but the principal route of elimination is via the kidney by a combination of glomerular filtration and tubular secretion. Accumulation occurs in renal impairment. Plasma half-life averages 2 hours. Most drugs in this group, such as enalapril and perindopril, are administered as prodrugs and require to be de-esterified in the liver to the active component. Elimination of ACE inhibitors is a function both of free drug clearance and binding to ACE, resulting in a biphasic half-life.

Dose–response relationships

As a general rule there is a close linear relationship between the plasma concentration of the active drug and the degree of ACE inhibition, and inversely with angiotensin II and aldosterone concentrations. The early decline in blood

Table 5.4 ACE inhibitors

ACE inhibitor	Active form	Elimination	T_{max} (h)	$T_{1/2}$ (h)	Duration of effect (h)
captopril		R	1	8	3–12
cilazapril	cilazaprilat	R	1	50	24
enalapril	enalaprilat	R	3	50	12–30
fosinopril	fosinoprilat	R:H 50:50	3	12	12–24
lisinopril		R	6	30	18–30
perindopril	perindoprilat	R	4	30	24
quinapril	quinaprilat	R	2		24
ramipril	ramiprilat	R	2	110	>24
trandolapril	trandolaprilat	R	4		24

pressure parallels the fall in plasma angiotensin II concentrations, but the long-term reduction in blood pressure bears no clear relationship to either the concentration of drug or to its effects on the renin–aldosterone axis.

Indications

ACE inhibitors are now accepted as first-line drugs in essential hypertension, although evidence from long-term morbidity/mortality studies is sparse. They are of similar broad efficacy to other main groups of antihypertensives (Treatment of Mild Hypertension Research Group, 1991), but are least effective in elderly Black patients (Materson *et al.*, 1993). The antihypertensive effect may be exaggerated when renin levels are increased, for example in renovascular hypertension, and when diuretics are co-administered.

The other main indication for ACE inhibitors is cardiac failure, where they now have a central role in management, improving pathophysiology, haemodynamics, symptoms and survival (Francis and McDonald, 1993; Packer, 1992). They are a clear first choice in elderly hypertensives with co-existing heart failure.

Many very large scale studies have also confirmed that ACE inhibitors have an important role after myocardial infarction (Ray *et al.*, 1993; Pfeffer, 1995). Unfortunately, they have not yet been shown to be of particular value in respect of primary prevention in uncomplicated hypertensives.

There is evidence to suggest that ACE inhibitors may be 'renoprotective' in diabetic patients with proteinuria (Lewis *et al.*, 1993). It has not yet been clearly established if this is a specific effect on glomerular function or whether this represents the outcome of improved blood pressure control, but the onus probably now lies with other antihypertensives to demonstrate equivalent efficacy in such patients.

Renovascular disease may be present in diabetics and any significant deterioration in renal function should prompt investigation of this possibility (Webster *et al.*, 1988).

Contraindications

There are few absolute contraindications to the use of ACE inhibitors in the elderly.

Hypersensitivity

Angio-oedema has been reported with a number of these drugs, and the probability is that this is a rare class effect. Re-exposure to any drug in the group would be inadvisable. Skin rashes also occur, but these are much less serious and it may be justified to observe the response to an alternative ACE inhibitor before abandoning the group.

Renal impairment

Severe deterioration in renal function may occur in patients with renal artery stenosis exposed to ACE inhibitors (Hollenberg, 1984; Hricik et al., 1983; Speirs et al., 1988). This is thought to result from failure of autoregulation within the nephron. In the presence of a critical renal artery stenosis, glomerular filtration in the affected kidney may be maintained by the constrictor effect of angiotensin II on efferent arteriolar tone. When the production of angiotensin II is inhibited by ACE inhibitors, glomerular filtration may plummet. This effect can be observed within 1 hour of administration of captopril and forms the basis of the captopril-enhanced renography test for functional stenosis (Ghione et al., 1985). At this stage the effect is reversible, but if treatment continues the kidney may cease to function and will atrophy. In patients with bilateral renal artery stenosis or with a stenosis affecting a solitary kidney, this effect may be manifest as a rise in serum creatinine (Silas et al., 1983). The time course for this may be days or months, or it may even occur years after the introduction of the drug as a result of progression of the underlying disease. If the disease is unilateral, no change in serum creatinine may be seen and the kidney may be unwittingly lost. Monitoring in either case poses considerable difficulties. This is a particular problem in the older patient as the prevalence of atheromatous disease affecting the aorta and renal arteries increases with age (Eyler et al., 1962).

Connective tissue disorders

When captopril was introduced into clinical practice in the late 1970s, a number of cases of neutropenia and proteinuria were reported (Cooper, 1983). It emerged that these appeared to be especially likely when the drug was used in patients with severe hypertension and renal impairment associated with scleroderma and systemic lupus erythematosus. As with many other antihypertensives, relatively high doses of the drug were used initially and this may partly explain the problem. Particular care must be taken if the drugs are used in such patients.

Adverse reactions

Hypotension

All ACE inhibitors may cause severe, symptomatic 'first dose' hypotension. Fortunately such instances are rare, particularly if a number of sensible clinical precautions are observed. Patients at particular risk are: the elderly (prone to the effects of hypotension through frailty, disequilibrium and cerebrovascular disease), patients with heart failure (often relatively hypotensive already), and renin-dependent patients (high dose diuretics, renovascular hypertension). In such patients it is wise to withhold diuretic therapy for 24 hours prior to introducing ACE inhibitors, starting with a very small dose and administering the first dose under supervision for the first 6 hours. In some patients this may require a brief hospital admission. For routine initiation in essential hypertension with none of these risk factors, it is sufficient to administer the first dose at bedtime, without the need for hospital supervision.

Renal impairment

As described above, all ACE inhibitors may induce a decline in renal function in the presence of renovascular disease. The time course is very variable. The result may be an insidious decline in the function of an affected kidney or the development of acute renal failure in the case of bilateral disease or a solitary functioning kidney. This effect may be accentuated by diuretic therapy or extracellular volume depletion.

Hypersensitivity

This problem is unpredictable but fortunately uncommon. Macular skin rashes typically affect the limbs and trunk. Angio-edema may relate to inhibition of breakdown of bradykinin, but is fortunately rare.

Cough

This is the commonest adverse effect of ACE inhibitors (Coulter and Edwards, 1987). It typically presents with a persistent dry, irritating, unproductive cough that usually troubles the patient at night and disturbs sleep. It is easily recognised in a previously asymptomatic hypertensive, but may be less easily attributed to the drug in a patient with heart failure who may have pre-existing cough. The frequency of this symptom is generally underestimated, but up to 15% of patients may be affected (Just, 1989). There is no unequivocal evidence that there are clinically important differences between different ACE inhibitors or that the cough can be ameliorated by NSAIDs or inhaled steroids or cromoglycate.

Taste disturbances have also been described with ACE inhibitors.

Drug interactions

Beneficial

In hypertension, ACE inhibitors may usefully be combined with all other major classes of antihypertensives.

Adverse

First dose hypotension and renal impairment are more likely if the patient is already on a diuretic. NSAIDs also increase the potential for adverse renal effects.

ACE inhibitors tend to conserve potassium and there is a risk of hyper-kalaemia if they are used in conjunction with potassium-sparing diuretics.

Major outcome studies

Many large trials now attest to the benefits of ACE inhibitors in heart failure (Francis *et al.*, 1993) and after myocardial infarction (Ray *et al.*, 1993).

ACE inhibitors seem to be as well tolerated and effective as most other major antihypertensive drug groups (Croog *et al.*, 1986; Materson *et al.*, 1993). To date, however, no large scale morbidity/mortality study has reported the use of ACE inhibitors as first-line therapy in hypertension.

ALPHA-BLOCKING DRUGS

Doxazosin, indoramin, prazosin and terazosin are second-line drugs in hypertension.

Mode of action

The predominant antihypertensive action of all of these drugs is competitive antagonism of peripheral post-junctional alpha$_1$-adrenoceptors. This action is highly selective. The dose–response curves to the alpha agonists, phenylephrine (exogenous) and noradrenaline (endogenous), are shifted in parallel to the right. Alpha-blockers have virtually no known adverse biochemical properties and this may be an advantage in some patients where there is concern about their renal function, liver function, or electrolyte status. There is some evidence of a beneficial effect on the lipid profile – total cholesterol is reduced by about 5%, triglycerides by up to 15% and high density lipoprotein increased by up to 10% (Weidmann *et al.*, 1985). However, this has never yet been shown to have been translated into clinical benefit and may be outweighed by the rather modest efficacy and unfavourable tolerability compared with other major antihypertensive drug groups.

Pharmacokinetics

All of these drugs are well absorbed, although the absorption of prazosin in particular is highly variable and subject to extensive 'first-pass' metabolism in the gut and liver. This is a considerable clinical disadvantage. Of the other drugs, the most satisfactory kinetic profile is that of doxazosin, with its reliable absorption and absence of significant 'first-pass' effect. All are extensively metabolised and the elimination half-lives range from 3 hours (prazosin) to 22 hours (doxazosin).

Dose–response relationships

There is no direct correlation between the dose of these drugs and the blood pressure response. Indeed, one of the principal problems with this group is unpredictable hypotension.

Indications

These drugs are indicated in hypertension, but only as second line when other drugs are contraindicated, poorly tolerated or ineffective. A number of additional indications do occasionally justify consideration of these drugs.

Heart failure

Prazosin is a combined arteriolar and venodilator and reduces cardiac preload and afterload. Preliminary studies suggested that it might benefit patients with heart failure (Colucci *et al.*, 1980), although there was some evidence that the beneficial effects of prazosin in this situation were not sustained. A subsequent large trial showed that prazosin was inferior to the combination of hydralazine and isosorbide (Cohn *et al.*, 1986), which combination in turn was shown to be inferior to enalapril (Cohn *et al.*, 1991).

Raynaud's phenomenon

Alpha-blockers have been used to alleviate symptoms in this frustrating condition, but earlier reports of benefit have not been borne out by large studies.

Prostatism

All of these drugs relax the outflow mechanism of the urinary bladder. In elderly men this property can be useful in alleviating the symptoms of benign prostatic hypertrophy (Chow *et al.*, 1990). This is especially useful if definitive surgery is contraindicated or deferred, and can usually be achieved without a major effect on blood pressure.

Contraindications

There are very few absolute contraindications to these drugs. True hypersensitivity would be but this is extremely rare.

Adverse reactions

The most notorious adverse effect of these drugs is 'first-dose' hypotension (Graham *et al.*, 1977). This has been a particular problem with prazosin, possibly as a result of incautious dosing but also relating to its rather unpredictable absorption and variable 'first-pass' metabolism. These drugs act as venodilators and the sudden reduction in venous filling that results may also contribute to this effect. If the problem were truly confined to the first dose this could to a very large extent be anticipated and catered for. However, patients frequently omit or forget to take tablets and the problem can recur each time the patient resumes their regular medication. In addition it may be accentuated by other antihypertensive drugs such as diuretics. Orthostatic hypotension may also occur with regular dosing. For these reasons, alpha-blockers are not recommended as first-line therapy in the older hypertensive, who may be particularly susceptible to such effects. If these drug are used it is essential to start with the lowest possible dose and titrate slowly upwards.

Other adverse effects relate to the effects of these drugs on the bladder neck sphincter. Urinary incontinence may occur, especially in older women in whom this can be a problem anyway, and ejaculatory failure has been reported in younger men. This may be offset against some benefits in older men with prostatism.

Other problems include weakness and fatigue, ankle oedema, and palpitations.

Intolerance is more common than with other major groups of antihypertensives (Materson *et al.*, 1993).

Major outcome studies

No major outcome trial has investigated the effect of alpha-blocking drugs in elderly hypertensives.

REFERENCES

Alderman EL, Coltart DJ, Wettach GE, Harrison DC 1974. Coronary artery syndromes after sudden propranolol withdrawal. *Annals of Internal Medicine* **81**, 625–7.
Amery A, Birkenhager W, Brixko P *et al.* 1985. Mortality and morbidity results from the European Working Party on High Blood Pressure in the Elderly trial. *Lancet* **1**, 1349–54.
Amery A, Birkenhager W, Bulpitt CJ *et al.* 1991. Syst-Eur. A multicentre trial on the treatment of isolated systolic hypertension in the elderly: Objectives, protocol, and organization. *Aging* **3**, 287–302.
Anderson J, Godfrey BE, Hill DM, Munro-Faure AD, Sheldon J 1971. A comparison of the effects of hydrochlorothiazide and frusemide in the treatment of hypertensive patients. *Quarterly Journal of Medicine* **40**, 541–60.
Anon 1991. Nifedipine. In Dollery CT (ed.) *Therapeutic drugs.* Edinburgh: Churchill Livingstone, N80–7.
Arieff AI 1986. Hyponatraemia, convulsions, respiratory arrest, and permanent brain damage after elective surgery in healthy women. *New England Journal of Medicine* **314**, 1529–35.
Ashraf N, Locksley R, Arieff AI 1981. Thiazide-induced hyponatraemia associated with death or neurological damage in outpatients. *American Journal of Medicine* **70**, 1163–8.
Atkinson AB, Cumming AMM, Brown JJ *et al.* 1982. Captopril treatment inter-dose variations in renin, angiotensins I and II, aldosterone and blood pressure. *British Journal of Clinical Pharmacology* **13**, 855–8.
Benson E, Webster J 1995. The tolerability of amlodipine in hypertensive patients. *British Journal of Clinical Pharmacology* **39**, 578P–9P.
Buhler FR, Laragh JH, Vaughan ED, Brunner HR, Gavras H, Baer L 1973. Antihypertensive action of propranolol. *American Journal of Cardiology* **32**, 511–22.

Bulpitt CJ, Fletcher AE, Amery A *et al*. 1994. The Hypertension in the Very Elderly Trial (HYVET). Rationale, methodology and comparison with previous trials. *Drugs and Aging* **5**, 171–83.

Buring JE, Glynn RJ, Hennekens CH 1995. Calcium channel blockers and myocardial infarction: a hypothesis formulated but not yet tested. *Journal of the American Medical Association* **274**, 654–5.

Burris JF, Weir MR, Oparil S 1990. An assessment of diltiazem and hydrochlorothiazide in hypertension. *Journal of the American Medical Association* **263**, 1507–12.

Carlsen JE, Kober L, Torp-Pedersen C 1990. Relation between dose of bendrofluazide, anti-hypertensive effect, and adverse biochemical effects. *British Medical Journal* **300**, 975–8.

Channer KS, McLean KA, Lawson-Matthew P, Richardson, M 1994. Combination diuretic treatment in severe heart failure: a randomised controlled trial. *British Heart Journal* **71**, 139–44.

Chow W, Hahn D, Sandhu D, Henshaw R, Das G, Wells P 1990. Multicentre controlled trial of indoramin in the symptomatic relief of benign prostatic hypertrophy. *British Journal of Urology* **65**, 36–8.

Cohn JN, Archibald DG, Ziesche S *et al*. 1986. Effect of vasodilator therapy on mortality in chronic congestive heart failure. Results of a Veterans Administration Cooperative Study. *New England Journal of Medicine* **314**, 1547–52.

Cohn JN, Johnson G, Ziesche S *et al*. 1991. A comparison of enalapril with hydralazine-isosorbide dinitrate in the treatment of chronic congestive heart failure. *New England Journal of Medicine* **325**, 303–10.

Colucci WS, Wynne J, Holman BL, Braunwald E 1980. Long term therapy of heart failure with prazosin. A randomized double blind trial. *American Journal of Cardiology* **45**, 337–44.

Committee on Safety of Medicines 1981. Timoptol eye drops. *Current Problems* **6**.

Coope JN, Warrender TS 1986. Randomised trial of treatment of hypertension in elderly patients in primary care. *British Medical Journal* **293**, 1145–51.

Cooper RA 1983. Captopril associated neutropenia, who is at risk? *Archives of Internal Medicine* **143**, 659–60.

Coulter DM, Edwards IR 1987. Cough associated with captopril and enalapril. *British Medical Journal* **294**, 1521–3.

Croog SH, Levine S, Testa MA *et al*. 1986. The effects of antihypertensive therapy on the quality of life. *New England Journal of Medicine* **314**, 1657–64.

Cruickshank JM 1981. Beta-blockers, bradycardia and adverse effects. *Acta Therapeutica* **7**, 309–21.

Cruickshank JM, Pritchard BNC 1988. *Beta-blockers in clinical practice*. Edinburgh: Churchill Livingstone, 275–433.

Dahlof B, Lindholm LH, Hannson L, Schersten B, Ekbom T, Wester P-O 1991. Morbidity and mortality in the Swedish Trial in Old Patients with Hypertension (STOP-Hypertension). *Lancet* **338**, 1281–5.

Davidson C, Thadani U, Singleton W, Taylor SH 1976. Comparison of antihypertensive activity of beta-blocking drugs during chronic treatment. *British Medical Journal* **2**, 7–9.

Davidson NMcD, Corrall RJ, Shaw TR, French EB 1977. Observations in man of hypogly-caemia during selective and non-selective beta-blockade. *Scottish Medical Journal* **22**, 69.

Deacon SP, Karunanayake A, Barnett D 1977. Acebutolol, atenolol, and propranolol and metabolic responses to acute hypoglycaemia in diabetes. *British Medical Journal* **2**, 1255–7.

Eyler WR, Clark MD, Garman JE, Rian RL, Meininger DE 1962. Angiography of the renal areas including a comparative study of renal arterial stenosis in patients with and without hypertension. *Radiology* **78**, 879–91.

Francis GS, McDonald K 1993. Overview of survival studies in left ventricular dysfunction. In Cleland JGF (ed.) *The clinician's guide to ACE inhibition*. Edinburgh: Churchill Livingstone, 150–63.

Fraunfelder FT, Barker AF 1984. Respiratory effects of timolol. *New England Journal of Medicine* **311**, 1441.

Furberg CD, Psaty BM, Meyer JV 1995. Nifedipine: dose related increase in mortality in patients with coronary heart disease. *Circulation* **92**, 1326–31.

Ghione S, Fommei E, Palombo C *et al*. 1985. Kidney scintigraphy after ACE inhibition in the diagnosis of renovascular hypertension. *Uraemia Investigation* **9**, 211–15.

Goldstein RE, Boccuzzi SJ, Cruess D, Nattel S and The Adverse Experience Committee and the Multicentre Diltiazem Post-infarction Research Group 1991. Diltiazem increases late-congestive heart failure in post infarction patients with early reduction in ejection fraction. *Circulation* **83**, 52–60.

Graham RM, Thornell IR, Gain JM, Bagnoli C, Oates J, Stokes GS 1977. A controlled study in hypertensive patients of the 'first dose phenomenon' observed with prazosin therapy. *Australian and New Zealand Journal of Medicine* **7**, 211–12.

Greenberg G, Brennan PJ, Miall WE 1984. Effects of diuretic and beta-blocker therapy in the Medical Research Council trial. *American Journal of Medicine* **76**(2A), 45–51.

Harron DWG, Balnave K, Kinney CD, Wilson R, Russell CJ, Shanks RG 1981. Effects on exercise tachycardia during 48 hours of a series of doses of atenolol, sotalol and metoprolol. *Clinical Pharmacology and Therapeutics* **29**, 295–302.

Hollenberg, NK 1984. Renal haemodynamics in essential and renal hypertension: influence of captopril. *American Journal of Medicine* **76**(5B), 22–8.

Horton R 1995. Spinning the risks and benefits of calcium antagonists. *Lancet* **346**, 586–7.

Hricik DE, Browning PJ, Kopelman R, Goorno WE, Madias NE, Dzau VJ 1983. Captopril-induced functional renal insufficiency in patients with bilateral renal artery stenosis or renal artery stenosis in a solitary kidney. *New England Journal of Medicine* **308**, 373–6.

Hugenholz PG, Rafflenbeul W, Hecker H, Jost S, Deckers JW and on behalf of the INTACT Group Investigators 1990. Retardation of angiographic progression of coronary artery disease by nifedipine (results of the International Nifedipine Trial on Anti-atherosclerotic Therapy (INTACT)). *Lancet* **335**, 1109–13.

IPPPSH Collaborative Group 1985. Cardiovascular risk and the risk factors in a randomized trial of treatment based on the beta-blocker oxprenolol: the International Prospective Primary Prevention Study in Hypertension (IPPPSH). *Journal of Hypertension* **3**, 379–92.

Isles CJ, Johnson AOC, Milne FJ 1986. Slow-release nifedipine and atenolol as initial treatment in blacks with malignant hypertension. *British Journal of Clinical Pharmacology* **21**, 377–83.

Israeli Sprint Study Group 1988. Secondary prevention reinfarction Israeli nifedipine trial (SPRINT). A randomized intervention trial of nifedipine in patients with acute myocardial infarction. *European Heart Journal* **9**, 354–64.

Jeffers TA, Webster J, Petrie JC, Barker NP 1977. Atenolol once-daily in hypertension. *British Journal of Clinical Pharmacology* **4**, 523–7.

Johnston GD, Wilson R, McDermott BJ, McVeigh GE, Duffin D, Logan J 1991. Low-dose cyclopenthiazide in the treatment of hypertension: a one year community- based study. *Quarterly Journal of Medicine* **78**, 135–43.

Just PM 1989. The positive association of cough with angiotensin-converting enzyme inhibitors. *Pharmacotherapy* **9**, 82–7.

Kloner RA 1995. Nifedipine in ischaemic heart disease. *Circulation* **92**, 1074–8.

Langman MJS, Weil J, Wainwright P *et al*. 1994. Risks of bleeding peptic ulcer associated with individual non-steroidal anti-inflammatory drugs. *Lancet* **343**, 1075–8.

Lewis EJ, Hunsicker IG, Bain RP, Rohde RD and for the Collaborative Study Group 1993. The effect of angiotensin-converting-enzyme inhibition on diabetic nephropathy. *New England Journal of Medicine* **329**, 1456–62.

Management Committee of the Australian National Blood Pressure Study 1980. The Australian therapeutic trial in mild hypertension. *Lancet* **2**, 1261.

Materson BJ, Reda DJ, Cushman WC *et al.* and Department of Veterans Affairs Cooperative Study Group on Antihypertensive Agents 1993. Single-drug therapy for hypertension in men. *New England Journal of Medicine* **328**, 914–21.

Medical Research Council Working Party 1992. Medical Research Council trial of treatment of hypertension in older adults: principal results. *British Medical Journal* **304**, 405–12.

Medical Research Council Working Party 1985a. MRC trial of treatment of mild hypertension: principal results. *British Medical Journal* **291**, 97–104.

Medical Research Council Working Party 1985b. MRC trial in mild hypertension: principal results. *British Medical Journal* **291**, 97–104.

Medical Research Council Working Party on Mild to Moderate Hypertension 1983. Ventricular extrasystoles during thiazide treatment: substudy of MRC mild hypertension trial. *British Medical Journal* **2**, 1249–53.

Morgan K 1993. The mechanism of ACE inhibitor action. In Cleland JGF (ed.) *The clinician's guide to ACE inhibition.* Edinburgh: Churchill Livingstone, 3–22.

Moser M 1989. Relative efficacy of, and some adverse reactions to, different antihypertensive regimens. *American Journal of Cardiology* **63**, 2B–7B.

Mullick FG, McAllister HA 1977. Myocarditis associated with methyldopa therapy. *Journal of the American Medical Association* **237**, 1699–1701.

Multicentre Dilthiazem Postinfarction Research Group 1988. The effect of dilthiazem on mortality and reinfarction after myocardial infarction. *New England Journal of Medicine* **319**, 385–92.

Opie LH, Messerli FH 1995. Nifedipine and mortality: grave defects in the dossier. *Circulation* **92**, 1068–73.

Packer M 1992. Treatment of chronic heart failure. *Lancet* **340**, 92–5.

Papademetriou V, Burris JF, Notargiacomo A, Fletcher RD, Freis ED 1988. Thiazide therapy is not a cause of arrhythmia in patients with systemic hypertension. *Archives of Internal Medicine* **148**, 1272–6.

Pfeffer MA 1995. ACE inhibition in acute myocardial infarction. *New England Journal of Medicine* **332**, 118–20.

Psaty BM, Heckbert SR, Koepsell TD *et al.* 1995. The risk of myocardial infarction associated with antihypertensive therapies. *Journal of the American Medical Association* **274**, 620–5.

Ray S, McMurray J, Dargie HJ 1993. ACE inhibition after myocardial infarction. In Cleland JGF (ed.) *The clinician's guide to ACE inhibition.* Edinburgh: Churchill Livingstone, 135–49.

Reid JL, Wing LMH, Dargie HJ, Hamilton CA, Davies DS, Dollery CT 1977. Clonidine withdrawal in hypertension: changes in blood pressure and in plasma and urinary noradrenaline. *Lancet* **1**, 1171–4.

Robb OJ, Webster J, Petrie JC and Harry J 1988. Effects of the beta²-adrenoceptor antagonist ICI 118551 on blood pressure in hypertensive patients known to respond to atenolol and propranolol. *British Journal of Clinical Pharmacology* **25**, 433–8.

Scognamiglio R, Rahimtoola SH, Fasoli G, Nistri S, Dalla Volta S 1994. Nifedipine in asymptomatic patients with severe aortic regurgitation and normal left ventricular function. *New England Journal of Medicine* **331**, 689–94.

Silas JH, Klenka Z, Solomon SA, Bone JM 1983. Captopril induced reversible renal failure: a marker of renal artery stenosis affecting a solitary kidney. *British Medical Journal* **286**, 1702–3.

Siscovick DS, Raghunathan TE, Psaty BM *et al.* 1994. Diuretic therapy for hypertension and the risk of primary cardiac arrest. *New England Journal of Medicine* **330**, 1852–7.

Speirs CJ, Dollery CT, Inman WHW, Rawson NSB, Wilton LV 1988. Postmarketing surveillance of enalapril. II: Investigation of the potential role of enalapril in deaths with renal failure. *British Medical Journal* **297**, 830–2.

Systolic Hypertension in the Elderly Program (SHEP) Cooperative Research Group 1991. Prevention of stroke by antihypertensive drug treatment in older patients with isolated systolic hypertension: final results of SHEP. *Journal of the American Medical Association* **265**, 3255–64.

Systolic Hypertension in the Elderly's Collaborative Group Co-ordinating Centre 1992. Systolic hypertension in the Elderly: Chinese trial (SYST-CHINA), interim report. *Chinese Journal of Cardiology* **20**, 270–5.

Toghill PJ, Smith PG, Benton P, Brown RC, Matthews HL 1974. Methyldopa liver damage. *British Medical Journal* **3**, 545–8.

Treatment of Mild Hypertension Research Group 1991. The Treatment of Mild Hypertension Study: a randomised, placebo-controlled trial of a nutritional-hygienic regimen along with various drug therapies. *Archives of Internal Medicine* **151**, 1413–23.

Weber MA 1980. Discontinuation syndrome following cessation of treatment with clonidine and other antihypertensive agents. *Journal of Cardiovascular Pharmacology* **2**(Suppl. 1), S73–89.

Webster J, Jeffers TA, Galloway DB, Petrie JC 1974. Withdrawal of antihypertensive therapy. *Lancet* **2**, 1318.

Webster J, Jeffers TA, Galloway DB, Petrie JC, Barker NB 1977. Atenolol, methyldopa and chlorthalidone in moderate hypertension. *British Medical Journal* **1**, 76–9.

Webster J, Murchison LEM, Robb OJ 1988. Angiotensin converting enzyme inhibitors may cause renal impairment in diabetes mellitus. *Scottish Medical Journal* **33**, 317–18.

Webster J, Petrie JC, Robb OJ, Jamieson M, Verschueren J 1985. A comparison of single doses of bucindolol and oxprenolol in hypertensive patients. *British Journal of Clinical Pharmacology* **20**, 393–400.

Webster J, Robb OJ, Witte K, Petrie JC 1987. Single doses of enalapril and atenolol in hypertensive patients treated with bendrofluazide. *Journal of Hypertension* **5**, 457–560.

Weidmann P, Uehlinger De, Gerber A 1985. Antihypertensive treatment and serum lipoproteins. *Journal of Hypertension* **3**, 297–306.

Wilcox RG, Hampton JR, Banks DC *et al.* 1986. Trial of early nifedipine in acute myocardial infarction: the TRENT study. *British Medical Journal* **293**, 1204–8.

Wilhelmson L, Berglund G, Elmfeldt D *et al.* and on behalf of the Heart Attack Primary Prevention in Hypertension Trial Research Group 1987. Beta-blockers versus diuretics in hypertensive men: main results from the HAPPHY trial. *Journal of Hypertension* **5**, 561–72.

Worlledge SM, Carstairs KG, Dacie JV 1966. Autoimmune haemolytic anaemia associated with alpha-methyldopa therapy. *Lancet* **2**, 135–9.

Yusuf S 1995. Calcium antagonists in coronary artery disease and hypertension. *Circulation* **92**, 1079–82.

CHAPTER 6

Ambulatory blood pressure in the elderly and blood pressure measurement

JOSEPH DUGGAN AND EOIN O'BRIEN ——————————————

INTRODUCTION

Accurate measurement of blood pressure in elderly subjects is essential, not only to ensure that those who are hypertensive and would benefit from treatment are diagnosed, but also to avoid treatment in those in whom it is not necessary, given the greater potential for side effects in this population. The accurate measurement of blood pressure presents particular problems that must be surmounted if satisfactory management is to be achieved. The purpose of this chapter is to put the difficulties of blood pressure measurement in the elderly into perspective, and to assess the role of ambulatory blood pressure measurement (ABPM) in diagnosis and management of hypertension in this age group.

CONVENTIONAL BLOOD PRESSURE MEASUREMENT IN THE ELDERLY

Blood pressure measurement in the elderly should not differ in principle from that in the population as a whole and standard recommendations, such as those of the British Hypertension Society, should be carefully followed (Petrie et al., 1986). However a number of aspects of blood pressure measurement in this age group warrant special consideration. First, blood pressure variability increases with age (Mancia et al., 1980; Parati et al., 1993). To avoid overdiagnosis, it is vital therefore to measure blood pressure on at least three different occasions and confirm sustained blood pressure elevation before making a diagnosis of hypertension. Second, selection of the correct bladder cuff is important for both conventional measurement and ABPM. Avoidance of undercuffing is important since it may lead to overestimation of blood pressure; however, in elderly patients lean arms are not uncommon and overcuffing with its attendant risk of underestimating blood pressure should be avoided (O'Brien et al., 1993b). Third, the occurrence of an auscultatory gap may be more common in the elderly. The

Korotkov sounds may initially be heard at the systolic blood pressure level, then disappear and become audible again at a level 30–35 mmHg below, finally disappearing completely at diastolic blood pressure levels. The underlying pathophysiological mechanism remains to be elucidated. The auscultatory gap is especially common in patients with isolated systolic hypertension, which would explain its greater prevalence in the elderly. Auscultation should begin with the cuff inflated to a level at least 20 mmHg above that at which the radial pulse disappears (Messerli and Schmeider, 1991). Blood pressure should also be checked in both arms since more than 10% of elderly patients have a greater than 10 mmHg difference in systolic pressure between arms (Fotherby *et al.*, 1993).

Spence and colleagues reported normal intra-arterial blood pressures in a group of elderly patients who were hypertensive according to conventional measurement (Spence *et al.*, 1978). It was suggested by Messerli and his colleagues that it was possible to distinguish between true hypertension and 'pseudohypertension' in these patients by the use of Osler's manoeuvre (Messerli *et al.*, 1985). Osler used the sign to detect 'sclerosis' of the vessel wall (Osler 1892). The manoeuvre is conducted by inflating the blood pressure cuff above systolic pressure, and, if the artery distal to the cuff is palpable, the sign is present. Arterial compliance was found to be lower in Osler-positive patients and the reduced compliance correlated with the difference between direct and indirect blood pressure indicating that the stiffer the artery the greater the degree of 'pseudohypertension' (Messerli *et al.*, 1985).

The prevalence of this condition in unselected elderly populations is probably less than originally thought. The extent to which a positive Osler sign predicts 'pseudohypertension' is open to question. To evaluate its importance in diagnosing pseudohypertension Oliner and colleagues (1993) investigated 19 hypertensive patients deemed Osler-positive by at least two observers. Blood pressure was determined indirectly by the conventional method and directly by a brachial artery catheter transducer monitoring system. Pseudohypertension was defined as a sphygmomanometric mean pressure that exceeded intra-arterial mean pressure by 10 mmHg or more. In this group of 19 Osler-positive patients, conventional sphygmomanometry underestimated systolic and overestimated diastolic intra-arterial pressure. Conventional measurement was 10 mmHg or more higher than intra-arterial pressure in two patients and 10 mmHg or more lower than intra-arterial pressure in three patients. While two patients had pseudohypertension, three appeared to have 'pseudohypotension', defined as a condition where indirect measurement significantly underestimates intra-arterial pressure. Therefore, a positive Osler's manoeuvre did not reliably predict the presence of pseudohypertension in this population. While the direct–indirect difference correlates with decreased compliance the percentage of variance attributable to decreased compliance is small at about 26% in normotensive elderly people (Finnegan *et al.*, 1985; Messerli *et al.*, 1985). Furthermore, there is little information on the prevalence of the sign in hypertension, and concordance between observers in eliciting the sign is potentially poor (Prochazka and Martel, 1987).

We have compared the accuracy of indirect blood pressure measurement in elderly hypertensive patients with that of younger patients (O'Callaghan *et al.*, 1983). Indirect measurement underestimated direct systolic pressure by 4.4 mmHg in the elderly and 7.0 mmHg in the young, and overestimated diastolic blood pressure by 9.2 mmHg and 10.4 mmHg, respectively. This study was conducted in consecutive patients attending our blood pressure clinic and led us to conclude that the standard technique for blood pressure measurement is as accurate in the elderly as it is in young patients. There may well be, however, a number of elderly hypertensive patients whose prevalence is unknown and who have a large disparity between direct and indirect blood pressure measurement. In such circumstances, conventional sphygmomanometry may overestimate both systolic and diastolic blood pressure. In such cases hypertension is correctly diagnosed but the severity is overestimated, therefore 'inappropriate hypertension' might be a better term than 'pseudohypertension'. A number of patients will, however, be misdiagnosed as hypertensive because their intra-arterial pressure is 'normal' whilst the cuff pressure is in the hypertensive range. Here the term 'pseudohypertension' is apposite (O'Brien and O'Malley, 1994).

Hypotension, particularly postural hypotension, may affect all age groups (Imholz *et al.*, 1990) but is particularly prevalent in the elderly, occurring in 20% of those in institutional care (Caird *et al.*, 1973) and in 10% of otherwise healthy elderly hypertensive subjects (Rodstein and Zeman, 1957). In a cross-sectional analysis of the 4736 participants in the SHEP study postural hypotension was assessed at 1 and 3 minutes after the patient arose from a seated position (Applegate *et al.*, 1991). Postural hypotension was found in 10.4% of participants at 1 minute and in 12% at 3 minutes. It was found that 5.3% of patients demonstrated postural hypotension at both time intervals whereas 17.3% demonstrated it at either or both time intervals. Higher mean systolic blood pressure and lower mean body-mass index were significantly associated with the presence of postural hypotension. They concluded that postural hypotension in healthy community-dwelling older people with isolated systolic hypertension (ISH), may not be associated with a history of disorders or problems usually considered to be related to postural hypotension. Prospective data are required to determine the prognostic significance of postural hypotension and whether one or multiple measurements carry more significance. Post-prandial hypotension is a frequently unrecognised phenomenon in the elderly. Blood pressure may fall by as much as 25 mmHg following a meal in elderly institutionalised patients (Lipsitz *et al.*, 1983). It is crucial therefore to measure blood pressure in the lying, standing and sitting positions, and to avoid recording blood pressure within 2 hours of meals (Haigh *et al.*, 1991).

AMBULATORY BLOOD PRESSURE MEASUREMENT (ABPM) IN THE ELDERLY

Non-invasive measurement of blood pressure in ambulatory humans began in the 1960s (Hinman *et al.*, 1962). Ambulatory devices have been modified over the years and are now pocket-sized with almost noiseless pumps. ABPM offers considerable advantages over conventional and invasive methods of blood pressure measurement and has now moved from the research arena into clinical practice. In this section the technical aspects of ABPM in the elderly will be considered and 'normal' ambulatory blood pressure levels in the elderly will be discussed. Furthermore, the role of ABPM in the diagnosis and management of hypertension in this age group will be evaluated.

Technical aspects of ABPM in the elderly

Since conventional blood pressure meaurement presents a problem in the elderly, it is not unreasonable to assume that automated devices will also have difficulty in recording accurate blood pressure levels. Few devices have been evaluated exclusively in elderly subjects. The accuracy of the TM-2420 ambulatory blood pressure monitor has been assessed in elderly subjects by Clark *et al.* (1992). They studied 94 subjects (44 men and 50 women), aged 60–94 with systolic blood pressures of 97–208 mmHg and diastolic blood pressures of 45–109 mmHg, including 23 patients with isolated systolic hypertension, in three centres. The monitor was compared simultaneously with pairs of observers using the Hawksley random zero sphygmomanometer. The standard deviation of the difference (SDD) between observers was 4.2 mmHg for systolic blood pressure and 2.9 mmHg for diastolic blood pressure. The mean difference was 0.49 mmHg and 0.27 mmHg, respectively, for systolic and diastolic blood pressure. The SDD between the monitor and the average of the observers' readings was 6.7 mmHg for systolic and 5.5 mmHg for diastolic blood pressure, with mean differences of 4.4 mmHg and 4.8 mmHg, respectively. There were no significant differences between the two versions of the monitor used (5 and 7) or between the three pairs of observers. The monitor was found to be equally accurate in isolated systolic hypertension. In a separate section of the study, a 24-hour ABPM was conducted using the device in 129 subjects aged 60–79 years. 89% of the monitorings attempted were successful with error rates of less than 10%. The device was well tolerated with only 4.7% of the subjects not completing a monitoring. The study does not, however, fulfill the criteria for validation according to the Association for the Advancement of Medical Instrumentation (AAMI) or the British Hypertension Society (BHS) protocols (O'Brien *et al.*, 1995). The AAMI protocol stipulates that a standard mercury sphygmomanometer should be used for comparison with the test device. The most serious protocol violation, which has occurred in eight studies, was substitution of the Hawksley random zero sphygmomanometer for the mercury sphygmomanometer (O'Brien *et al.*, 1995). This was done with the intention of reducing observer bias but the Hawksley has subsequently been shown to underestimate blood pressure (O'Brien *et al.*, 1990a) and the effect this may have on validation studies has been discussed in detail by Conroy and his colleagues (1993). In a further study, these authors combined a database of paired blood pressure measurements using the Hawksley random zero sphygmomanometer and a standard mercury sphygmomanometer, and a database of paired measurements made on a SpaceLabs 90202 ambulatory recorder and standard sphygmomanometer, to determine how the SpaceLabs 90202 would have fared if it had been assessed against the Hawksley random zero sphygmomanometer instead of a standard sphygmomanometer. The effect of replacing the standard instrument with a Hawksley sphygmomanometer was to reverse the direction of the average measurement error found and to demote the SpaceLabs 90202 from BHS grades C and B, for systolic and diastolic accuracy respectively, to grade D overall; the lowest rating of accuracy in the BHS grading system (Conroy *et al.*, 1994). The conclusions of validation studies using the Hawksley sphygmomanometer as to the accuracy or otherwise of the device being validated are, therefore, questionable (O'Brien *et al.*, 1995).

There is some evidence that device accuracy deteriorates in older subjects (Miller *et al.*, 1992). Miller and his colleagues compared simultaneous measurements from the Accutracker II ambulatory monitor and from two trained observers who ausculatated blood pressure simultaneously in the same arm in the conventional manner, using a stethoscope and mercury sphygmomanometer, in 103 subjects ranging in age from 23 to 92 years. The difference between the Accutracker II and the mercury standard averaged 6 mmHg for both systolic and diastolic pressures. However, these results must again be viewed with some caution because of the questionable accuracy of the device used. The discrepancy between the Accutracker II and the mercury standard was systematically related to certain characteristics of the participants. Systolic blood pressure correlated significantly with age, gender and race with age showing the strongest correlation. For persons younger than 50 years of age, systolic blood pressure was 2.0 mmHg lower when measured by ABPM; however, for persons over 50 years of age the difference in measurements between techniques was 8.3 mmHg. For those over 70 years of age, this difference had increased to 11 mmHg. When the effect of blood pressure level on the discrepancy between the techniques was examined, 31% of the variance between the techniques was attributed to age and blood pressure level, of which 17% was due to a joint effect resulting from correlation between age and level of blood pressure, 4.5% to age alone, and 9.4% to blood pressure level alone. If the criteria of the AAMI were applied to these results, the Accutracker II would fail to fulfill the accuracy requirement of this standard (American National Standard, 1987). These findings are consistent with an earlier validation study performed according to the AAMI criteria (O'Brien *et al.*, 1991a).

These results suggest that ambulatory systems for use in the elderly should be evaluated specifically in an aged population and that the effects of age and blood pressure level on accuracy should be carefully examined. Until validation studies are conducted specifically in elderly subjects, we must rely on the validation studies done in samples from the general population and use the most accurate devices for ABPM in the elderly (O'Brien *et al.*, 1993c).

We have shown that device accuracy also worsens with increasing blood pressure levels (O'Brien *et al.*, 1993a). We validated six ambulatory systems according to the British Hypertension Society protocol (O'Brien *et al.*, 1993d). During the performance of these validation studies, a tendency was noted for accuracy to deteriorate with increasing levels of blood pressure. Further analysis was conducted, therefore, to examine the accuracy of these six ambulatory systems, not only across the blood pressure range recommended in the BHS protocol but also in low (<130/80 mmHg), medium (130/80 to 160/100 mmHg), and high (>160/100 mmHg) blood pressure ranges (O'Brien *et al.*, 1993c). When the data was analysed according to tertiles of pressure for low, medium and high pressure ranges, all six devices held their overall rating or improved slightly in the low and medium pressure ranges. In the high pressure range, however, the rating of all six devices deteriorated. These results suggest that all six ambulatory devices are less accurate in subjects whose blood pressure at entry to the validation study was above 160/100 mmHg. This finding has important implications since ambulatory blood pressure measuring devices are used most often in clinical practice to determine diagnosis or to assess the efficacy of antihypertensive drug treatment in patients whose blood pressures may be in the range in which these devices are least accurate, a situation that may be particularly likely in the elderly. It must be emphasised, however, that experience in interpreting data for pressure ranges is limited, and the number of subjects included for analysis is necessarily considerably less than that used for the overall analysis. Although it would be preferable to have 85 patients in each tertile of blood pressure range, the feasibility of doing such a validation is daunting, and we believe that the trend towards deteriorating accuracy in the higher pressure ranges is one that potential users and manufacturers should recognise. Furthermore, the original AAMI (American National Standard, 1987) and BHS (O'Brien *et al.*, 1993d) validation procedures may mask the important influence of pressure level on device accuracy. The BHS protocol has addressed this issue in the revised version (O'Brien *et al.*, 1993d).

In choosing an ambulatory system, consideration should be given to the accuracy of the device in measuring the levels of blood pressure likely to be encountered in the population being studied. Since high blood pressures, particularly systolic blood pressures, may be encountered in the elderly, careful consideration should be given to the available validation data before using ambulatory systems (O'Brien *et al.*, 1993c). When accuracy is required accross the whole pressure range, it would seem from tertile analysis that the CH-Druck and SpaceLabs 90207 are the most accurate. However, available information on device accuracy in elderly subjects is limited and the BHS, in its revised protocol for validating blood pressure measuring systems, has devoted a sub-section to validation of devices in the elderly (O'Brien *et al.*, 1993d).

Ambulatory blood pressure measurement levels in a normal population

A number of population studies to determine normal reference values for ABPM have been published (O'Brien, 1994). Reference tables for different nationalities demonstrating normal levels for different ages and gender have been produced. A meta-analysis of data from 19 studies conducted in Europe, the USA, the Far East and Australia has been performed by Staessen and his colleagues (1993). The major disadvantage of such studies is that the 'normalcy' of the population is dependent on inclusion and exclusion criteria and selection, in any event, is based on conventional blood pressure. Notwithstanding this, sufficient evidence has accumulated to allow a good 'working' definition of normal ABPM by age and sex. For example, in the Allied Irish Bank (AIB) study, using the mean +/− 2 standard deviations as the upper limit of normal, values are obtained for 24-hour pressure of 140/86 mmHg, 148/94 mmHg for daytime pressure and 128/77 mmHg for night-time pressure in subjects in whom the upper limit of normal for office pressure was 149/96 mmHg (O'Brien *et al.*, 1991b). In the meta-analysis by Staessen and colleagues (1993), the pooled estimate of the mean plus two standard deviations in normotensive persons was 139/87 mmHg for the 24-hour pressures and 146/91 and 127/79 mmHg, respectively, for the daytime and night-time pressures. Using the data from these studies allows us to produce, with some confidence, a working definition of normalcy which would have 140/90 mmHg as the upper limit of normal for 24-hour pressure, 150/95 mmHg for daytime pressure and 130/80 mmHg for night-time pressure (O'Brien and Staessen, 1995). With regard to the effect of age, the 95th centiles for daytime ambulatory pressure in men were 114/88 mmHg for the 17–29-year age group and 155/103 mmHg in those aged 50–79 years with corresponding levels in women of 131/83 mmHg and 177/97 mmHg (O'Brien *et al.*, 1991b). It is evident, therefore, that there are considerable differences for age and gender for which allowance must be made. Furthermore, normal values for ABPM in the very elderly (those aged over 80 years) are not available and we are currently conducting a population study in this age group.

ABPM in diagnosis and management of hypertension in the elderly

Conventional versus ABPM

The fact that blood pressure varies throughout the day in all age groups is well recognised; therefore office blood pressure is limited in that the reading obtained may not be representative of the patient's blood pressure in the long term. Potential sources of observer error, either systematic error, terminal digit preference or observer prejudice, or sphygmomanometer innaccuracy, may limit reliability of conventional measurement and have been extensively reviewed (O'Brien and O'Malley, 1991a). ABPM removes observer error, reduces white-coat effect and provides blood pressure readings throughout the day (Duggan, 1994). The reproducibility of ambulatory measurements is superior to that of conventional measurements in the general population (Coats, 1990) and specifically in the elderly (Engfeldt *et al.*, 1994; Fotherby and Potter, 1993). Fotherby and Potter (1993) compared the reproducibility of clinic and ambulatory blood pressure measurements in elderly hypertensive subjects. They investigated 22 untreated elderly hypertensives with a clinic systolic pressure greater than 160 mmHg and/or diastolic blood pressure greater than 95 mmHg. Patients were aged 66–86 years with a mean age of 76 years. Following three supine clinic blood pressure readings the subjects underwent 24-hour ABPM, with measurements at 20-minute intervals from 07.00 to 22.00 h and at 30-minute intervals from 22.00 to 07.00 h. Measurements were repeated during a further visit at a median interval of 10 weeks. The mean 24-hour ambulatory systolic and diastolic blood pressure reproducibility, which was assessed by the standard deviation of the differences between visits, was significantly better than that for mean clinic blood pressure. They concluded that both 24-hour and daytime ABPM significantly improved the reproducibilty of blood pressure measurements compared with clinic blood pressure readings in elderly hypertensive subjects. Increasing the number of daytime readings by 50% (from 30 to 45) reduced the variability of blood pressure measurement by 50%. They concluded that more than 30 readings were needed during a daytime recording to significantly reduce variability compared with repeated clinic measurements. However, night-time variability was not significantly altered if the number of measurements was reduced to 12 over a 6-hour period.

Engfeldt and colleagues (1994) investigated the reproducibility of 24-hour ABPM in elderly normotensive individuals at baseline and after 1 year. They randomly selected 34 subjects; 10 were aged 65 years, 10 were aged 70 years, eight were aged 75 years, and six were aged 80 years. The Spacelabs 90207 monitor was used and one baseline and one follow-up ABPM 1 year later was conducted. A mean of 97% of the measurements were successful and only two of the 34 subjects were excluded because of measurement failures. The standard deviations of the differences between the baseline and 1 year measurements were 8/4 mmHg and 12/8 mmHg for daytime and night-time respectively. They concluded that ABPM is readily accepted as a clinical investigation in normotensive elderly subjects and that the reproducibility of ABPM after 1 year is good.

Blood pressure variability in the elderly

The fact that blood pressure is continuously changing from minute to minute is not a recent finding. In fact the first description of blood pressure variability was by Hales in 1733. Since then many investigators have emphasised the continuous variability of blood pressure over time. Commonly available devices for ABPM do not permit assessment of blood pressure variability that requires blood pressure to be continuously monitored on a beat to beat basis. Until recently, this type of recording was only possible if invasive intra-arterial monitoring was used. New devices that offer a non-invasive system for continuous ABPM have now been developed (Imholz *et al.*, 1993). This system, which uses small cuffs wrapped around two fingers permits monitoring of the beat to beat blood pressure changes triggered, for example, by laboratory stimuli. In a preliminary validation study in which continuous intra-arterial blood pressure monitoring was compared with the Portapres finger monitoring device, it was found that the Portapres device was capable of reliably monitoring the blood pressure changes that occurred throughout a 24-hour period (Imholz *et al.*, 1993).

To date, however, the changes in blood pressure variability over a 24-hour period that occur with age have been defined using continuous intra-arterial blood pressure monitoring. Variability of systolic blood pressure was found to increase with ageing and the nocturnal fall in blood pressure was reported to be less pronounced (Mancia *et al.*, 1983; Rowlands *et al.*, 1984). Furthermore, the variability in heart rate was reduced with age. The reduced heart rate variability may reflect the reduced parasympathetic modulation of the heart that occurs with age (Ferrari *et al.*, 1991), whereas the increased blood pressure variability may reflect both an increased arterial stiffness and reduced neural homeostatic mechanisms with ageing. The increased blood pressure variability may well have important clinical implications in determining the rate of cardiovascular complications in the elderly. In fact, a greater degree of end-organ damage in hypertensive patients has been reported in those with increased variability of their 24-hour blood pressure in addition to those with a reduced night-time fall in blood pressure (Parati *et al.*, 1992; Verdecchia *et al.*, 1990).

Detailed analysis of blood pressure and heart rate variability, in both the time and frequency domain, provides important insights into neural control of the circulation (Parati *et al.*, 1993). In the time domain, analysis of the transient increases or decreases in systolic blood pressure associated with reciprocal changes in heart rate which occur spontaneously over 24 hours provides a method to dynamically evaluate baroreflex modulation of the heart (Parati *et al.*, 1988). Information from this type of analysis implies that the sensitivity of baroreflex control of heart rate is significantly impaired with age. In fact, not only is there a reduction in the average 24-hour baroreflex sensitivity, but also there is a loss of the normal physiological increase at night-time (Parati *et al.*, 1993). These changes are similar to the changes that occur in hypertension.

Due to their augmented blood pressure variability and reactivity, inaccuracies in isolated office blood pressure readings are exaggerated in the elderly. The correlation between office and ambulatory blood pressure is lower in the elderly than in younger subjects (Khoury *et al.*, 1992), which may reflect the increased lability of blood pressure in the elderly. As stated previously, a number of features of the 24-hour blood pressure profile are altered with ageing. As quantified by the standard deviation of the 24-hour average value, elderly subjects as compared with young controls have a higher degree of overall variability in systolic blood pressure and a lower variability in 24-hour heart rate (Khoury *et al.*, 1992; Mancia *et al.*, 1983). The increased overall variance in systolic blood pressure over the entire 24-hour period, however, has been reported to be associated with a reduced amplitude of its day to night fluctuations (Khoury *et al.*, 1992). The likelihood of an erroneous overestimation of actual blood pressure and subsequent unnecessary antihypertensive drug treatment is increased in this age group if conventional measurement alone is used (Parati *et al.*, 1993), and this suggests a potential 'special' role for assessment of hypertension in this age group.

White-coat hypertension

The discrepancy between clinic and home blood pressure presents an important clinical problem as to which is the most representative of the 'true' blood pressure level. The true pressure may be taken as the average pressure over a prolonged period of time and appears to be a more important predictor of target organ damage than clinic pressure (O'Brien, 1994). 24-hour ABPM provides the best means of answering this question. Pickering and colleagues (1982) compared clinic and ambulatory blood pressures in three groups of subjects: normotensive subjects and patients with borderline or established hypertension. In both groups of hypertensive patients the average clinic pressures were higher than the average 24-hour levels, but in the normotensive subjects there was no difference between clinic and ambulatory levels. It is often stated that clinic pressure represents the patient's response to everyday stresses, but this has been refuted by Pickering and his colleagues (1988). This group could find no difference between white-coat hypertensive and sustained hypertensive patients in terms of either variability of blood pressure on ABPM or the blood pressure response to stress as evidenced by the difference between home and work blood pressures. White-coat hypertension may be defined as a persistently elevated clinic blood pressure with normal blood pressure at other times. As for other types of hypertension the precise definition tends to be arbitrary. Pickering's group (1988) have used a cut-off point of 90 mmHg for the clinic pressure based on the fact that this is the most widely accepted level. ABPM is used to establish that the blood pressure is normal outside the clinic and a cut-off for the upper limit of normal is defined. They have chosen the 90th percentile of the daytime blood pressure on ambulatory monitoring as the upper limit, which was 134/90 mmHg, based on recordings in 37 normal subjects. To be classified as having white-coat hypertension their patients had to have daytime pressures below these levels in conjunction with elevated clinic pressure.

When discussing white-coat hypertension it is important to establish definitions to avoid confusion (Fig. 6.1). We propose that the term 'white-coat hypertension' should be reserved for those patients who exhibit elevated office blood pressures that settle within a short time to give normal daytime mean blood pressure (Fig. 6.2), and that the term 'white-coat effect' should be reserved for those patients who exhibit elevated office blood pressures that fall with ABPM but do not lower the mean daytime blood pressure to normal (Fig. 6.3) (O'Brien and O'Malley, 1994).

In younger and middle-aged patients white-coat hypertension occurs with a prevalence of approximately 20% (Pickering *et al.*, 1988). Pickering found that 21% of patients with borderline hypertension (clinic diastolic pressures between 90 and 104 mmHg) had both systolic and diastolic pressures that were below this level during ABPM. In contrast, patients with more severe hypertension (clinic diastolic pressure above 105 mmHg) had a much lower prevalence of white-coat hypertension of 5%. Others have reported similar findings. In one study, 60 patients with mild hypertension were investigated, all of whom had been advised to take antihypertensive medication on the basis of clinic blood pressure (Krakoff *et al.*, 1988). The average clinic pressure was 155/100 mmHg and the average ambulatory pressure was 131/82 mmHg with 38% having ambulatory pressures below 130/85 mmHg. Although different criteria were used (clinic

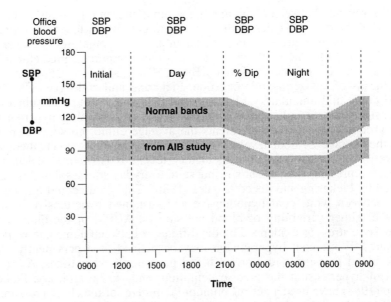

Fig. 6.1   Scheme for the presentation of the data described in the remaining figures in this chapter. The 24-hour period is divided into four windows: the white-coat window during the first hour of recording when blood pressure may be elevated due to the white-coat effect; the daytime window; the nocturnal window; and the percentage nocturnal dip in blood pressure. The systolic and diastolic blood pressures (SBP; DBP) for each of these windows are printed across the top of the plot. The shaded bands indicate the upper and lower limits of blood pressure as derived from the Allied Irish Bank Study

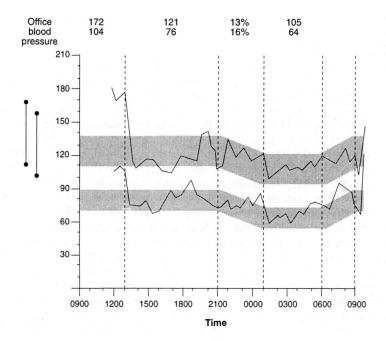

Fig. 6.2   White-coat hypertension

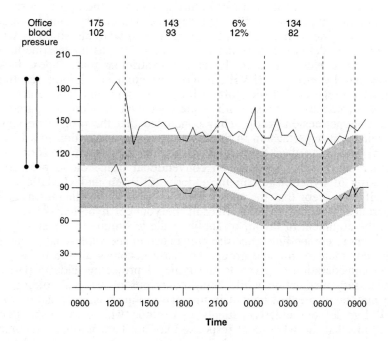

Fig. 6.3   White-coat effect

systolic or diastolic pressure at least 10 mmHg higher than daytime ambulatory pressures) a prevalence of 39% in a clinic population of 98 patients was reported (Lerman *et al.*, 1989).

White-coat hypertension may have a higher prevalence in older patients. In patients over the age of 60 years who were being screened for the Systolic Hypertension in the Elderly Program (SHEP), the prevalence of white-coat hypertension was 42% (Ruddy *et al.*, 1988). In this study, the clinic and ambulatory pressures of 81 patients with systolic hypertension were compared with age-matched normotensive subjects, all of whom were aged 60 years or more. 42% of those with clinic systolic hypertension had ambulatory pressures in the normotensive range. Others have also reported that this phenomenon is commoner in the elderly (Lerman *et al.*, 1989). Shimada and colleagues (1990b) investigated the pressor response to blood pressure measurement in a routine outpatient setting in 104 elderly hypertensive patients. Blood pressure was measured at 5-minute intervals before, during and after the visit using ABPM. The average rise in systolic and diastolic pressures upon a patient's visit to the doctor's room was 17 and 7 mmHg, respectively. There was an associated tachycardia and the increase in systolic blood pressure was more pronounced in female compared with male patients. Blood pressure and heart rate returned to the baseline level approximately 40 minutes after leaving the doctor's office. In a population of 50 untreated hypertensive patients aged 70 years or over, Trenkwalder and colleagues (1993) conducted ABPM, ECG and echocardiography to assess the frequency of white-coat hypertension. White-coat hypertension was diagnosed if mean daytime ambulatory blood pressure was less than, or equal to, 146/87 mmHg (taken as the upper 'normal' limit), and definite hypertension if mean daytime ambulatory blood pressure was greater than 146/87 mmHg. Nine patients (18%) were classified as white-coat, 28 (56%) as definite hypertensives and 13 (26%) as an intermediate group. Lower office blood pressure, lower left ventricular mass index, lack of left ventricular hypertrophy (LVH), a more pronounced alerting reaction and a lack of correlation between office blood pressure and left ventricular mass (LVM) characterised those with white-coat hypertension compared with the definite hypertension group. They concluded that the prognostic significance of white-coat hypertension in the elderly requires evaluation in a larger population. Taken together, these studies raise the important question as to how much reliance can be placed on conventional office blood pressures in the diagnosis of hypertension in the elderly (O'Brien and O'Malley, 1994). In fact, if we accept that the most effective method for diagnosing white-coat hypertension and white-coat effect in the younger hypertensive is by ABPM, then the argument in favour of applying the technique to the elderly becomes all the more compelling since the prevalence of the white-coat phenomenon is more common in this age group. The case becomes all the more persuasive when consideration is given to the issue of protecting elderly patients from unnecessary medication while being conscious of not withholding treatment that may be of greatest benefit in this age group. It is our practice to perform ABPM in all our elderly patients to exclude white-coat responders, while accepting that the white-coat response may not be a normal phenomenon but one which merits continuing observation but not necessarily antihypertensive medication.

Assessment of nocturnal blood pressure

In both normotensive and hypertensive subjects, the normal diurnal pattern of blood pressure involves a decrease of 10 to 20% during the hours of sleep (Pickering, 1993). If daytime is defined as 06.00–22.00 h and night-time as 22.00–06.00 h, and those hypertensive patients with a nocturnal reduction in average daytime systolic and diastolic blood pressure of less than 10% are classed as non-dippers, the prevalence of non-dippers in essential hypertension would appear to be in the order of 35% (Verdecchia *et al.*, 1991). In women (but not men), LVM seemed to be greater in non-dippers than dippers. To test this hypothesis, 24-hour ABPM and echocardiography were conducted in 260 hypertensive patients and 63 healthy normotensive subjects (Verdecchia *et al.*, 1992). LVM did not differ between dippers and non-dippers in hypertensive men; however, in hypertensive women it was significantly lower in dippers than non-dippers. In hypertensive women there was an inverse correlation between LVM and the percentage reduction of systolic and diastolic blood pressures from day to night, but this relationship did not exist in hypertensive men. These investigators concluded that, compared with men, hypertensive women require a longer duration of exposure to elevated blood pressure levels during the 24-hour period before developing LVH. More recently the same group of researchers investigated the hypothesis that an association exists between a blunted or absent nocturnal fall in blood pressure and future cardiovascular morbid events in patients with essential hypertension (Verdecchia *et al.*, 1993). This was a case control study. The case subjects were 32 hypertensive subjects with a first fatal or non-fatal major cardiovascular event, who had had ABPM conducted, but who had been off anti-hypertensive therapy for 1 to 5 years. Control subjects were 49 hypertensive patients free from cardiovascular events. Analysis of the baseline ambulatory blood pressure profile revealed that for men the nocturnal reductions of blood pressure did not differ between cases and controls; however, for women the nocturnal reductions in blood pressure were significantly less in cases than in controls. They concluded from this retrospective case control study, that there was an association between the reduction or absence of the usual nocturnal fall in blood pressure and future cardiovascular events in women with hypertension (Verdecchia *et al.*, 1993).

The diurnal blood pressure pattern may well be altered with age; however, there is no consensus in the literature. In the Allied Irish Bank study of normotensive subjects, age did not appear to influence diurnal blood pressure (O'Brien *et al.*, 1991b). In hypertensive patients, similar diurnal patterns were found in those aged above and below 55 years (Drayer *et al.*, 1983). In a study of 133 hypertensive and 91 normotensive subjects, no age-related change in the amplitude of the diurnal blood pressure rhythm was present, although the amplitude of the heart rate rhythm reduced with age (Munkata *et al.*, 1991). On the other hand, the nocturnal fall of systolic but not diastolic blood pressure was reported to be less pronounced in hypertensive subjects over the age of 65 years as compared with younger subjects (Khoury *et al.*, 1992). More recently, in a study of 31 hypertensive patients aged 25–74 years, Atkinson and colleagues (1994) reported a significant age-related reduction in the amplitude of the circadian rhythms in systolic blood pressure and heart rate. In contrast, elderly patients with isolated systolic hypertension are reported to have greater nocturnal falls of both systolic and diastolic pressures than age-matched normotensive or diastolic hypertensive subjects but without differences in the diurnal rhythm of heart rate. In summary, therefore, there is a lack of consensus with regard to the influnce of age on diurnal blood pressure and further studies are necessary.

On the other hand, there is growing evidence that hypertensive patients whose nocturnal blood pressure declines, so-called 'dippers', have less cardiovascular damage and consequent risk than the minority of patients whose blood pressure fails to fall at night, 'non-dippers' (O'Brien *et al.*, 1988; Pickering, 1990). A small number of studies have reported findings in elderly patients. A higher prevalence of target organ damage, either LVH or disease of the major arteries, was found in non-dippers than dippers in a small study of 14 elderly patients (Kobrin *et al.*, 1984). Kuwajima and colleagues (1992) investigated circadian blood pressure changes using ABPM in two groups of elderly hypertensive patients, those with and without LVH. 15 patients with LVH, 23 patients without LVH and 11 normotensive elderly subjects were studied. Although the daytime systolic blood pressure was comparable in the two hypertensive groups, the night-time SBP tended to be higher in patients with LVH than those without LVH. The LVM index correlated significantly with the night-time systolic pressure but not with the day-time pressure, clinic systolic pressure, or the systolic pressure following handgrip exercise. The difference in the systolic blood pressure between daytime and night-time in patients with LVH was significantly less than in patients without LVH. Furthermore, the difference between daytime and night-time systolic pressure correlated inversely with the LVM index. They concluded that hypertension in elderly patients with LVH is associated with a diminished nocturnal decline in blood pressure. Shimada and colleagues (1990a) initially reported that the extent of 'silent' cerebrovascular disease (measured as lacunae on a magnetic resonance image) in elderly hypertensive patients was more closely related to ambulatory than clinic pressure. More recently, this group has reported that the nocturnal blood pressure was more closely related to brain damage than was the daytime pressure, with greater changes being found in non-dippers than dippers (Shimada *et al.*, 1992).

Perhaps of greater relevance in the elderly as compared with the young is the possibility that excessive lowering of nocturnal blood pressure by critically altering perfusion of vital organs may predispose to cardiac and cerebral ischaemic events (O'Brien and O'Malley, 1994). It is reasonable to assume that the elderly, in whom cardiovascular haemodynamics may be compromised, are more susceptible to cerebrovascular events consequent upon excessive reduction of nocturnal blood pressure due to inordinate antihypertensive medication. Such an occurrence would be especially likely in elderly hypertensive patients who exhibit a pronounced nocturnal dipping pattern (Fig. 6.4). Since nocturnal blood pressure can only be characterised by 24-hour ABPM, this should be performed routinely to avoid excessive blood pressure lowering at night.

Hypotension

The problem of postural hypotension has been referred to earlier and, using conventional measurement, unless blood pressure is taken in the three recommended positions these patients may appear hypertensive. A characteristic pattern may appear using ABPM, particularly in those with severe postural hypotension

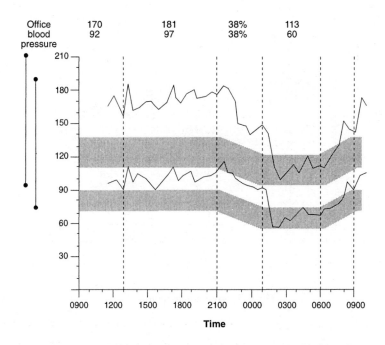

Fig. 6.4   Daytime hypertension with large nocturnal dipping pattern

secondary to autonomic failure with daytime hypotension and nocturnal hypertension (Fig. 6.5). Clearly, the administration of antihypertensive medication to
such patients could be disadvantageous and ABPM is proving to be a valuable
technique in assessing this group of patients and also in those with post-prandial
hypotension (Zachariah *et al.*, 1991).

Isolated systolic hypertension

ISH is a common condition in the elderly occurring in 8% of those aged 60–69
years and increasing to 22% of those aged 80 years or more (SHEP, 1993). These
percentage estimates translate into a daunting reality that nearly 4 million
Americans aged 60 and older have ISH and are likely to be considered for treatment. However these statistics derive from conventional measurement and
whilst there is no denying the risk of ISH (Kannel and Brand, 1985), perhaps not
all patients with ISH require treatment.
    Silagy and colleagues (1990) demonstrated that in a small number of elderly
patients with ISH, mean ambulatory blood pressures were consistent with that
diagnosis for only 8% of the daytime period. In another study it was shown that
there was a marked discrepancy between clinic and daytime pressures in patients
with ISH, with the former being some 27 mmHg higher than ambulant pressures
(Cox *et al.*, 1991). These results have been confirmed in the preliminary analysis
of the ambulatory side-project of the Syst-Eur study (Staessen *et al.*, 1992). In a
further study, Silagy and colleagues (1992) compared repeated clinic blood

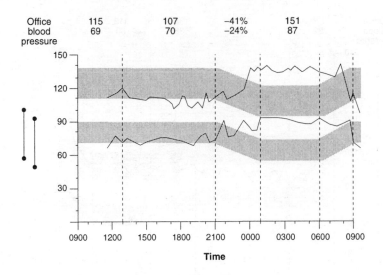

Office	115	107	–41%	151
blood	69	70	–24%	87
pressure				

Fig. 6.5   Autonomic failure

pressure measurement with ABPM in 10 elderly subjects with ISH and 11 normotensive controls. Mean clinic blood pressure was consistently higher than
mean daytime ambulatory blood pressure in both clinical groups and the effect
was greater for systolic than diastolic pressure and in the ISH group than the normotensive group. In the ISH group, the frequency distribution of systolic pressure readings was shifted to the right, whereas the distribution of diastolic
readings overlapped that of the normotensive group. They concluded that a
pressor response may explain the elevated systolic blood pressure observed in
elderly subjects with sustained ISH found on casual blood pressure measurement. Taken together, these studies suggest that ISH is not always a sustained
phenomenon, and, in many patients, the observed rise in office pressure is a manifestation of the alerting reaction (Silagy *et al.*, 1993). There are, therefore, two
forms of ISH on ABPM, 'sustained' ISH and 'transient' ISH (Figs 6.6 and 6.7).
One might postulate that antihypertensive medication could be targeted at those
elderly patients with sustained ISH. However, such a recommendation awaits
published evidence that cardiovascular risk is predicted more accurately by
ABPM than conventional measurement.

An accumulating body of evidence indicates that ambulatory pressures corre-
late more closely than clinic pressures with several different indices of target
organ damage (Pickering and Devereux, 1987). In a preliminary analysis of ambulatory measurements of blood pressure carried out in the run-in phase of the ambulatory monitoring side-project of the SYST-EUR study, the association between
left ventricular size (determined by ECG voltage criteria) and blood pressure
(assessed by clinic measurements) and ABPM was investigated in 97 elderly
patients. The additional diagnostic precision conferred by ABPM on clinic blood
pressure measurement was assessed by relating the residual ambulatory blood
pressure level to the ECG-left ventricular size. The residual ambulatory blood

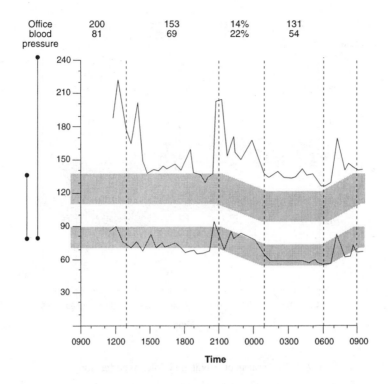

Fig. 6.6 'Sustained' isolated systolic hypertension

pressure level was calculated by subtracting the predicted ambulatory blood pressure level for each patient from the observed ambulatory blood pressure. Clinic systolic pressure was on average 20 mmHg higher than daytime ambulatory blood pressure whereas diastolic pressure was similar with both techniques. ECG voltage was significantly related to clinic systolic pressure, 24-hour, daytime and night-time ambulatory pressure levels. The ECG voltage was also significantly related to the residual ambulatory blood pressure levels. Therefore, ECG voltage criteria correlated more closely with ABPM than with office blood pressure, suggesting that ABPM is a better predictor of LVH than clinic measurement in elderly patients with ISH (Cox *et al.*, 1993). The ongoing side-project on ABPM in the SYST-EUR study should establish whether these findings hold true for morbidity and mortality. Until such information becomes available, ABPM should be used in elderly patients with ISH to identify those with sustained elevation who may require drug treatment and those in whom ISH is not sustained. For the latter, the decision to treat may be influenced by additional factors, such as the presence of end-organ damage (O'Brien and O'Malley, 1994).

ABPM in clinical practice

ABPM is being introduced into clinical practice at a rapid pace. In at least six European countries, ambulatory monitors have become available in general

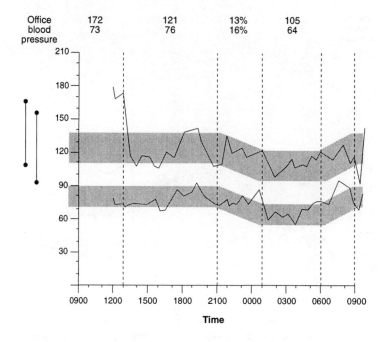

Fig. 6.7   'Transient' isolated systolic hypertension

practice. Market rather than scientific considerations may influence the introduction of a new development into clinical practice and the pharmaceutical companies are prominent in propagating ABPM in general practice. It is now very
clear that ABPM is passing from the research arena to clinical practice and it is
imperative that adequate guidelines are provided to avoid misuse. A number of
basic criteria must be fulfilled.

Device and operator requirements

Ambulatory systems must be accurate, reasonably priced and the recorders
should be noiseless, compact, light and comfortable to wear. A cuff with an
appropriate sized bladder should be used in those with obesity. It is essential
that the operator be experienced in the use of the equipment and understands
the normal ranges of blood pressure and the factors that might affect the diurnal pattern. The operator should be familiar with calibration of the monitor
and carefully instruct the patient to allow a maximum number of recordings
during the 24-hour period. Patients themselves must be able to contend with
the monitor and look after it carefully. It is important that the conditions of
measurement be standardised; the arm should be held still during measurement; similar levels of activity should be undertaken on recording days, if
recordings are to be compared, and for shift-workers, similar shifts should be
compared (Pickering *et al.*, 1991). In clinical practice, recordings are usually

programmed every 30 minutes. Subjects should keep a diary of activities during the recording period, although it is expected that motion-logging devices will soon be available to provide an objective assessment of activity (Van Egeren, 1991).

The indications for ABPM in clinical practice can be considered in terms of the diagnosis of hypertension and the selection and evaluation of antihypertensive drug treatment.

Diagnosis

A more accurate diagnosis of hypertension is possible using ABPM. Normalcy over a 24-hour period can be determined, white-coat hypertension can be excluded, borderline hypertension and dipper status can be identified.

Normalcy

Since normal ranges for ABPM have been defined according to gender and age, it is possible to assess whether the 24-hour blood pressure profile of a particular patient lies within the normal bands using either two standard deviations or the 5th and 95th centiles to indicate the upper and lower limits of pressure.

White-coat hypertension

Blood pressure elevation due to the white-coat effect is most effectively diagnosed using ABPM, thereby potentially avoiding treatment in 20% of patients with elevated office pressures.

Borderline hypertension

ABPM plays an important role in patients with borderline hypertension by helping to decide whether subjects with borderline elevation of office blood pressure should be labelled hypertensive. The finding of a normal ABPM profile may help to avoid the associated insurance costs of being labelled hypertensive. Furthermore, in those borderline hypertensives with target organ damage but normal ABPM, it is possible to exclude hypertension as the cause.

Dipper status

ABPM allows patients whose blood pressure does not fall at night (non-dippers) to be identified. These patients may need more careful evaluation to exclude a secondary cause of hypertension, and careful blood pressure control because of the potentially greater risk of target organ damage and morbidity previously alluded to.

Other areas of diagnostic use

ABPM is proving useful in diagnosis and assessment of patients with orthostatic hypotension, in identifying transient hypertension in phaeochromocytoma and in diagnosis of hypertension in subgroups such as Blacks, children and pregnant women (O'Brien, 1994).

ABPM in the selection and evaluation of antihypertensive drug treatment

Selection of drug and dosage regimen

With the advent of 24-hour ambulatory monitoring it is now possible to select a drug suited to the individual's blood pressure profile rather than relying on conventional measurement at a particular time point that may simply reflect the relationship between the time of measurement and the time of administration of the drug. Different classes of antihypertensive drugs may have differing effects on the circadian rhythm of blood pressure; therefore, certain drugs may be more suitable to patients with a particular 24-hour blood pressure profile. The results of one retrospective study indicate that hypertensive patients treated with beta-blockers sustain a significantly smaller nocturnal dip than untreated hypertensives, angiotensin-converting enzyme inhibitor-treated patients have accentuated blood pressure dipping compared to those taking beta-blockers and those treated with diuretics or calcium channel blockers have similar nocturnal dipping to untreated patients (Stanton *et al.*, 1990). In patients with an accentuated dip, therefore, one might choose a shorter acting drug or one with little effect on nocturnal pressure. In contrast, drugs with proven effect on nocturnal pressure might be prescribed in non-dippers.

Detecting white-coat responders

The ability of 24-hour monitoring to exclude those with white-coat hypertension from unnecessary treatment is an important advance and has major implications for the patients themselves and in terms of massive financial savings (Krakoff *et al.*, 1991). Raccaud and colleagues (1992) investigated the hypothesis that elderly in common with younger hypertensive patients tend to be overtreated if therapeutic decisions are based exclusively on office blood pressure measurements. They investigated 18 hypertensive patients aged 70 years or more who had office systolic blood pressures greater than or equal to 170 mmHg and/or diastolic blood pressures greater than or equal to 100 mmHg. The physicians caring for these patients were instructed to reduce blood pressure within 4 months to a target of less than or equal to 160/95 mmHg using any drug regimen. ABPM was conducted but the results were not available to the participating physicians until the conclusion of the study. At baseline, 11 patients had mean daytime ambulatory pressures less than 170/100 mmHg. Those patients whose blood pressure was elevated only in the doctor's presence did not have a reduction in their ambulatory pressure when antihypertensive therapy was initiated or intensified in order to reduce office blood pressure. This contrasted with the significant fall in ambulatory blood pressure observed in the presence of the doctor. They concluded that ABPM was useful in avoiding overtreatment not only of younger but also of elderly hypertensive patients.

Drug efficacy

24-hour monitoring proves to be a superior method to conventional measurement in evaluating efficacy of a given drug and is particularly useful in assessing pressure control in those patients with persistently raised office measurements. It is also useful in identifying those with an excessive blood pressure reduction, who may be at risk of myocardial infarction (Alderman *et al.*, 1989).

ABPM in the evaluation of antihypertensive efficacy of new agents

ABPM has played an important role in the evaluation of new antihypertensive agents for many years. The advantages of ABPM over conventional measurement in this setting may be considered in relation to the ability of the technique to detect drug effects which may not be evident with conventional measurement, to provide information on the duration of antihypertensive drug efficacy, and the ability to demonstrate the effect of drugs on nocturnal blood pressure and to detect the potential problems associated with excessive lowering of blood pressure. It is important to observe not only the efficacy of blood pressure reduction in studies of antihypertensive drugs, but also the the magnitude of this reduction, the leese of pressure, as we have termed it (O'Brien and O'Malley, 1991b).

One of the most surprising aspects of research into the efficacy of antihypertensive drugs is the readiness with which a blood pressure-lowering effect observed at one moment in the 24-hour cycle, often without reference to the time of drug administration, has been taken to indicate therapeutic efficacy throughout the day. With the increasing use of new formulations of drugs that permit once- and twice-daily dosage it is now more important than ever to be able to assess the pattern as well as the duration of drug effect (O'Brien *et al.*, 1989).

ABPM provides what was previously obtainable only with direct invasive intra-arterial measurement; an assessment of antihypertensive drug effect over 24 or 48 hours. Until recently interest in this aspect of ABPM centred on the desirability of being able to demonstrate that a drug was efficacious for the appropriate period related to dosing. ABPM has a number of features that allow for improvement in the design of antihypertensive drug studies: detection (and exclusion) of white-coat responders, simplification of the study design by virtue of a small or absent placebo response, lack of regression to the mean, thereby permitting selection of subjects with elevated blood pressure which will not fall with time, and finally the increased number of measurements provided by the technique permit recruitment of fewer subjects for antihypertensive drug studies.

There is some evidence that different groups of antihypertensive drugs may perturb the circadian pattern of blood pressure in different ways. Hypertensive patients on ACE inhibitors were shown in one study to have had markedly accentuated systolic and diastolic dipping patterns compared to untreated hypertensives and patients on beta-blockers, whereas hypertensive patients treated with beta-blockers, calcium channel blockers or diuretics had similar diastolic and systolic dipping patterns to the untreated groups (NHBPEP, 1990). Whatever the explanation for these varying effects of different groups of antihypertensive agents, which must be assessed in more detail in prospective studies, the fact that some drugs may accentuate nocturnal dipping, that others may blunt the normal nocturnal fall in blood pressure and that others have no effect on diurnal rhythmicity, raises important questions in assessing antihypertensive drug effect and in choosing a drug for an individual patient.

CONCLUSION

Elderly patients with hypertension present a challenge to the diagnostic and management skills of the physician. On the one hand there is the crucial issue of diagnosis. Is the patient truly hypertensive? Because of the white-coat phenomenon and the realisation that ISH may be simply an office phenomenon in many patients, ABPM becomes an essential investigation for accurate diagnosis in the elderly. Furthermore there are the idiosyncratic aspects of blood pressure behaviour in the elderly, such as ISH, increased blood pressure variability and autonomic dysfunction, each of which can be categorised more accurately with ABPM than with conventional measurement. With regard to treatment of the elderly hypertensive patient, ABPM can prove a useful adjunct to conventional measurement. It allows selection of the most appropriate antihypertensive drug for the individual patient given the diurnal pattern of blood pressure, thereby avoiding administration of excessive therapy during periods of endogenous blood pressure lowering, such as during sleep. In the assessment of the common manifestastions of hypotension in the elderly, ABPM permits the association of actual blood pressure levels with symptoms. If we are to conclude that ABPM should be used routinely in the assessment of elderly patients with apparent hypertension on conventional measurement, we must emphasise the need to carefully select devices of proven accuracy in this age group.

Finally, the relationship of ABPM to end-organ damage is the subject of ongoing studies, which serves as a reminder that blood pressure, whether measured conventionally or by ABPM, is only one aspect of the elderly patient's cardiovascular profile. Assessing target organ disease by echocardiography or other means permits an assessment of the impact of blood pressure on the cardiovascular system, which is ultimately likely to determine prognosis.

REFERENCES

Alderman M, Ooi W, Madhavan S, Cohen H 1989. Treatment-induced blood pressure reduction and the risk of myocardial infarction. *Journal of the American Medical Association* **262**, 920–4.

American National Standard 1987. Electronic or Automated Sphygmomanometers. Association for the Advancement of Medical Instrumentation, Arlington, VA.

American National Standard 1993. Electronic or Automated Sphygmomanometers. Association for the Advancement of Medical Instrumentation, Arlington, VA.

Applegate W, Davis B, Black H, Smith W, Miller S, Burlando A 1991. Prevalence of postural hypotension at baseline in the Systolic Hypertension in the Elderly Program (SHEP) cohort. *Journal of the American Geriatrics Society* **39**, 1057–64.

Atkinson G, Witte K, Nold G, Sasse U, Lemmer B 1994. Effects of age on circadian blood pressure and heart rate rhythms in patients with primary hypertension. *Chronobiology International* **11**, 35–44.

Caird FI, Andrews GR, Kennedy RD, 1973. Effect of posture on blood pressure in the elderly. *British Heart Journal* **35**, 527–30.

Clark S, Fowlie S, Pannarale G, Bebb G, Coats A 1992. Age and blood pressure measurement: experience with the TM2420 ambulatory blood pressure monitor and elderly people. *Age and Ageing* **21**, 398–403.

Coats AJS 1990. Reproducibility or variability of casual and ambulatory blood pressure data: implications for clinical trials. *Journal of Hypertension* **8**(Suppl. 6), S17–20.

Conroy R, Atkins N, Mee F, O'Brien E, O'Malley K 1994. Using Hawksley random zero sphygmomanometer as a gold standard may result in misleading conclusions. *Blood Pressure* **3**, 283–6.

Conroy R, O'Brien E, O'Malley K, Atkins N 1993. Measurement error in the Hawksley random zero sphygmomanometer: What damage has been done and what can we learn? *British Medical Journal* **306**, 1319–22.

Cox J, Amery A, Clement D *et al.* 1993. Relationship between blood pressure measured in the clinic and by ambulatory monitoring and left ventricular size as measured by electro-cardiogram in elderly patients with isolated systolic hypertension. *Journal of Hypertension* **11**, 269–76.

Cox J, Atkins N, O'Malley K, O'Brien E 1991. Does isolated systolic hypertension exist on ambulatory blood pressure measurement? *Journal of Hypertension* **9**(Suppl. 6), S100–1.

Drayer J, Weber M, DeYoung J, Wyle F 1983. Circadian blood pressure patterns in ambula-tory hypertensive patients: effects of age. *American Journal of Medicine* **72**, 493–9.

Duggan J 1994. Ambulatory blood pressure monitoring. *Pharmacology and Therapeutics* **63**.

Engfeldt P, Danielsson B, Nyman K, Aberg K, Aberg H 1994. 24 hour ambulatory blood pressure monitoring in elderly normotensive individuals and its reproducibility after one year. *Journal of Human Hypertension* **8**, 545–50.

Ferrari A, Daffonchio A, Gerosa S, Mancia G 1991. Alterations in cardiac parasympathetic function in aged rats. *American Journal of Physiology* **260**, 647–9.

Finnegan TP, Spence JD, Wong DG, Wells GA 1985. Blood pressure measurement in the elderly: Correlation of arterial stiffness with differences between intra-arterial and cuff pressures. *Journal of Hypertension* **3**, 231–5.

Fotherby M, Potter J 1993. Reproducibility of ambulatory and clinic blood pressure measurements in elderly hypertensive subjects. *Journal of Hypertension* **11**, 573–9.

Fotherby MD, Panayiotou B, Potter JF 1993. Age related differences in simultaneous inter-arm blood pressure measurements. *Postgraduate Medical Journal* **69**, 194–6.

Haigh RA, Harper GD, Burton R, Macdonald IA, Potter JF 1991. Possible impairment of the sympathetic nervous system response to postprandial hypotension in elderly hyper-tensives. *Journal of Human Hypertension* **5**, 83–9.

Hales S 1733. Haemastaticks. In Hales S (ed.) *Statistical essays*. London: Innys & Mauby, 1–186.

Hinman AT, Engel BT, Bickford AF 1962. Portable blood pressure recorder. Accuracy and preliminary use in evaluating intradaily variations in pressure. *American Heart Journal* **63**, 663–8.

Imholz B, Dambrink J, Karemaker J, Wieling W 1990. Orthostatic circulatory control in the elderly evaluated by non-invasive continuous blood pressure measurement. *Clinical Science* **79**, 73–9.

Imholz B, Langewouters G, van Montfrans G 1993. Feasibility of ambulatory, continuous 24-hour finger arterial pressure recording. *Hypertension* **21**, 65–73.

Kannel W, Brand F 1985. Cardiovascular risk factors in the elderly. In Andreas R, Bierman E, Hazzard W (eds) *Principles of geriatric medicine*. New York: McGraw-Hill, 104–19.

Khoury S, Yarows S, O'Brien T, Sowers J 1992. Ambulatory blood pressure monitoring in a nonacademic setting: effect of age and sex. *American Journal of Hypertension* **5**, 616–23.

Kobrin I, Dunn G, Oigman W 1984. Essential hypertension in the elderly: circadian varia-tion of arterial pressure. In Weber M, Drayer J (eds) *Ambulatory blood pressure monitor-ing*. Darmstadt: Steinkopff, 181–6.

Krakoff L, Eison H, Phillips R, Leiman S, Lev S 1988. Effect of ambulatory pressure moni-toring on the diagnosis and cost of treatment for mild hypertension. *American Heart Journal* **116**, 1152–4.

Krakoff L, Schechter C, Fahs, M, Andre M 1991. Ambulatory blood pressure monitoring; is it cost effective? *Journal of Hypertension* **9**(Suppl. 8), S28–30.

Kuwajima I, Suzuki Y, Shimosawa T 1992. Diminished nocturnal decline in blood pressure in elderly hypertensive patients with left ventricular hypertrophy. *American Heart Journal* **67**, 1307–11.

Lerman C, Brody D, Hui T 1989. The white-coat hypertension response: Prevalence and predictors. *Journal of General Internal Medicine* **4**, 226–31.

Lipsitz LA, Nyquist R, Wei J, Rowe JW 1983. Postprandial reduction in blood pressure in the elderly. *New England Journal of Medicine* **309**, 81–3.

Mancia G, Ferrari A, Gregorini L 1980. Blood pressure variability in man: its relation to high blood pressure, age and baroreflex sensitivity. *Clinical Science* **59**, 401–4.

Mancia G, Ferrari A, Gregorini L 1983. Blood pressure and heart rate variabilities in normotensive and hypertensive human beings. *Circulation Research* **53**, 96–104.

Messerli F, Ventura H, Amodeo C 1985. Oslers manoeuvre and pseudohypertension. *New England Journal of Medicine* **312**, 1548–51.

Messerli H, Schmeider R 1991. Blood pressure measurement in the elderly. In O'Brien E, O'Malley K (eds) *Blood pressure measurement.* Birkenhager WH, Reid JL, series eds, *Handbook of hypertension.* Amsterdam: Elsevier, 148–54.

Miller S, Elam J, Graney M, Applegate B 1992. Discrepancies in recording systolic blood pressure of elderly persons by ambulatory blood pressure monitor. *American Journal of Hypertension* **5**, 16–21.

Munkata M, Imai, Y, Abe K 1991. Assessment of age-dependent changes in circadian blood pressure rhythm in patients with essential hypertension. *Journal of Hypertension* **9**, 407–15.

National High Blood Pressure Education Program (NHBPEP) 1990. *Working group report on ambulatory blood pressure monitoring.* US Department of Health and Human Services. Public Health Service. National Institutes of Health, National Heart, Lung, and Blood Institute. Bethesda, MD. US NIH Publication No. 90–3028.

O'Brien E 1994. Blood pressure measurement. In Swales J (ed.) *Textbook of hypertension.* Oxford: Blackwell Scientific Publications, 989–1008.

O'Brien E, Atkins N, Mee F, O'Malley K 1993a. Comparative accuracy of six ambulatory devices according to blood pressure levels. *Journal of Hypertension* **11**, 672–5.

O'Brien E, Atkins N, O'Malley K 1993b. Selecting the correct bladder according to the distribution of arm circumference in the population. *Journal of Hypertension* **22**, 1149–50.

O'Brien E, Atkins N, Sheridan J 1991a. Evaluation of the Accutracker II non-invasive ambulatory blood pressure recorder according to the AAMI standard. *Journal of Ambulatory Monitoring* **4**, 27–33.

O'Brien E, Atkins N, Staessen J 1995. State of the market: a review of ambulatory blood pressure measuring devices *Hypertension* **26**, 835–42.

O'Brien E, Cox J, O'Malley K 1989. Ambulatory blood pressure measurement in the evaluation of blood pressure lowering drugs. *Journal of Hypertension* **7**, 243–7.

O'Brien E, Mee F, Atkins N, O'Malley K 1990a. Inaccuracy of the Hawksley random zero sphygmomanometer. *Lancet* **336**, 1465–8.

O'Brien E, Mee F, Atkins N, O'Malley K 1993c. Technical aspects of ambulatory blood pressure monitoring in the elderly. *Cardiology in the Elderly* **1**, 464–9.

O'Brien E, Murphy J, Tyndall A *et al.* 1991b. Twenty-four-hour ambulatory blood pressure in men and women aged 17 to 80 years: the Allied Irish Bank Study. *Journal of Hypertension* **9**, 355–60.

O'Brien E, O'Malley K 1991a. Clinical blood pressure measurement. In Birkenhager WH, Reid J (eds) *Handbook of hypertension*, Vol. 15. Amsterdam: Elsevier.

O'Brien E, O'Malley K 1991b. Ambulatory blood pressure monitoring in the evaluation of antihypertensive drug efficacy. *American Heart Journal* **121**, 999–1006.

O'Brien E, O'Malley K 1994. Blood pressure measurement in the elderly with special reference to ambulatory blood pressure measurement. In Leonetti G, Cuspidi C (eds), *Hypertension in the elderly*. Netherlands: Kluwer, 13–25.

O'Brien E, Petrie J, Littler W 1990b. The British Hypertension Society Protocol for the evaluation of automated and semi-automated blood pressure measuring devices with special reference to ambulatory systems. *Journal of Hypertension* **8**, 607–19.

O'Brien E, Petrie J, Littler W 1993d. The British Hypertension Society Protocol for the evaluation of blood pressure measuring devices. *Journal of Hypertension* **11**(Suppl. 2), S43–63.

O'Brien E, Sheridan J, O'Malley K 1988. Dippers and non-dippers. *Lancet* **ii**, 397.

O'Brien E, Staessen J 1995. Normotension and hypertension as defined by 24-hour ambulatory blood pressure monitoring. In Joan Ocon-puyadas (ed.) *Ambulatory Blood Pressure Monitoring*.

O'Callaghan W, Fitzgerald D, O'Malley K, O'Brien E 1983. Accuracy of indirect blood pressure measurement in the elderly. *British Medical Journal* **286**, 1545–6.

Oliner C, Elliot W, Gretler D, Murphy M 1993. Low predictive value of positive Osler manoeuvre for diagnosing pseudohypertension. *Journal of Human Hypertension* **7**, 65–70.

Osler W 1892. *Principles and practice of medicine*. New York: Appleton-Century.

Parati G, Di Rienzo M, Bertinieri G 1988. Evaluation of the baroreceptor-heart rate reflex by 24-hour intra-arterial blood pressure monitoring in humans. *Hypertension* **12**, 214–22.

Parati G, Di Rienzo M, Mancia G 1993. Ambulatory blood pressure monitoring in the elderly: evaluation of antihypertensive treatment and analysis of blood pressure variability. *Cardiology in the Elderly* **1**, 474–82.

Parati G, Omboni S, Di Rienzo M 1992. Twenty-four hour blood pressure variability: clinical implications. *Kidney International* **41**(Suppl. 37), S24–8.

Petrie J, O'Brien E, Littler W, deSwiet M 1986. Recommendations on blood pressure measurement. *British Medical Journal* **293**, 611–15.

Pickering T 1990. The clinical significance of diurnal blood pressure variations; dippers and non-dippers. *Circulation* **19**, 93–101.

Pickering T 1993. Clinical value of ambulatory blood pressure measurement in the elderly. *Cardiology in the Elderly* **1**, 490–3.

Pickering T, Devereux R 1987. Ambulatory monitoring of blood pressure as a predictor of cardiovascular risk. *American Heart Journal* **114**, 925–8.

Pickering T, Harshfield G, Kleinert H, Blank S, Laragh J 1982. Blood pressures during normal daily activities, sleep, and exercise. Comparison of values in normal and hypertensive subjects. *Journal of the American Medical Association* **247**, 992–6.

Pickering TG, James GD, Boddie C, Harshfield GA, Blank S, Laragh JH 1988. How common is white coat hypertension? *Journal of American Medical Association* **259**, 225–8.

Pickering T, Schnall P, Schwartz J, Pieper C 1991. Can behavioural factors produce a sustained elevation of blood pressure? Some observations and a hypothesis. *Journal of Hypertension* **9**(Suppl. 8), S66–8.

Prochazka A, Martel R 1987. Oslers manoeuvre in outpatients veterans. *Journal of Clinical Hypertension* **3**, 554–8.

Raccaud O, Waeber B, Petrillo A 1992. Ambulatory blood pressure monitoring as a means to avoid overtreatment of elderly hypertensive patients. *Gerontology* **38**, 99–104.

Rodstein M, Zeman F 1957. Postural blood pressure changes in the elderly. *Journal of Chronic Disease* **6**, 581–8.

Rowlands B, Stallard T, Littler W 1984. Continuous ambulatory monitoring of blood pressure and assessment of cardiovascular reflexes in the elderly hypertensive. *Journal of Hypertension* **2**, 615–22.

Ruddy MC, Bialy GB, Malka E, Lacy CR, Kostis JB 1988. The relationship of plasma renin activity to clinic and ambulatory blood pressure in elderly people with isolated systolic hypertension. *Journal of Hypertension* **6**(Suppl. 4), S412–15.

Shimada K, Kawamoto A, Matsubayashi K 1992. Diurnal blood pressure variations and silent cerebrovascular damage in elderly patients with hypertension. *Journal of Hypertension* **10**, 875–8.

Shimada K, Kawamoto A, Matsubayashi K, Ozawa T 1990a. Silent cerebrovascular disease in the elderly: correlation with ambulatory blood pressure. *Hypertension* **16**, 692–9.

Shimada K, Ogura H, Kawamoto A, Matsubayashi K, Ishida H, Ozawa T 1990b. Noninvasive ambulatory blood pressure monitoring during clinic visit in elderly hypertensive patients. *Clinical and Experimental Hypertension Theory and Practice* **12**, 151–70.

Silagy C, McNeill J, Farish S, McGrath B 1993. Comparison of repeated measurement of ambulatory and clinic blood pressure readings in isolated systolic hypertension. *Clinical and Experimental Hypertension* **15**, 895–909.

Silagy C, McNeill J, McGrath B 1990. Isolated systolic hypertension: Does it really exist on ambulatory blood pressure monitoring? *Clinical and Experimental Pharmacology and Physiology* **17**, 203–6.

Silagy C, McNeill J, McGrath B, Farish S 1992. Is isolated systolic hypertension a white coat phenomenon in the elderly? *Clinical and Experimental Pharmacology and Physiology* **19**, 291–3.

Spence J, Sibbald W, Cape R 1978. Pseudohypertension in the elderly. *Clinical Science* **55**(Suppl. 4), 399–402.

Staessen J, Amery A, Clement D 1992. Twenty-four hour blood pressure monitoring in the Syst-Eur trial. *Aging Clinical Experimental Research* **4**, 85–91.

Staessen J, O'Brien E, Atkins N, Amery A 1993. The ambulatory blood pressure in normotensive and hypertensive subjects. *Journal of Hypertension* **11**, 1289–97.

Stanton AV, Atkins N, O'Malley K, O'Brien E 1990. Circadian blood pressure and antihypertensive drugs. *American Journal of Hypertension* **3**, 107A.

Systolic Hypertension in the Elderly Program (SHEP) Cooperative Research Group 1993. Implications of the Systolic Hypertension in the Elderly Program. *Hypertension* **21**, 335–43.

Trenkwalder P, Plaschke M, Steffes-Tremer I, Lydtin H 1993. White-coat hypertension and alerting reaction in elderly and very elderly hypertensive patients. *Blood Pressure* **2**, 262–71.

Van Egeren L 1991. Monitoring activity and blood pressure. *Journal of Hypertension* **9**(Suppl. 8), S25–7.

Verdecchia P, Gatteschi C, Benemio G 1990. Circadian blood pressure changes and left ventricular hypertrophy in essential hypertension. *Circulation* **81**, 528–36.

Verdecchia P, Schillaci G, Boldrini F, Guerrieri M, Porcellati C 1992. Sex, cardiac hypertrophy and diurnal blood pressure variations in essential hypertension. *Journal of Hypertension* **10**, 683–92.

Verdecchia P, Schillaci G, Gatteschi C *et al.* 1993. Blunted nocturnal fall in blood pressure in hypertensive women with future cardiovascular morbid events. *Circulation* **88**, 986–92.

Verdecchia P, Schillaci G, Porcellati C 1991. Dippers versus non-dippers. *Journal of Hypertension* **9**(Suppl. 8), S42–4.

Zachariah P, Krier J, Schwartz G 1991. Orthostatic hypotension and ambulatory blood pressure monitoring. *Journal of Hypertension* **9**(Suppl. 8), S78–80.

CHAPTER 7

Non-pharmacological treatments for hypertension in the older adult

PR JACKSON, WW YEO AND LE RAMSAY ————————————

INTRODUCTION

The prospect of lowering blood pressure by methods other than drug therapy is appealing, especially in elderly subjects who have an incidence of sustained hypertension as high as 60% (Whelton *et al.*, 1993). A small downward shift in population blood pressure achieved by universal implementation of non-pharmacological measures might move a large number of the elderly below the level requiring drug treatment. In addition, a proportion of the many strokes and heart attacks which occur in those whose blood pressure is generally considered 'normal' may be prevented. For those who do need treatment for hypertension, non-pharmacological measures could improve blood pressure control or reduce the requirements for drugs.

The evidence on non-pharmacological treatments is imperfect for many reasons, and is even less satisfactory in relation to elderly patients. Evaluation of non-pharmacological management of hypertension often falls below the standards required when investigating antihypertensive drugs. The effect of non-pharmacological measures on blood pressure is generally small, and large numbers of subjects are therefore needed to confirm efficacy. For this reason many of the intervention trials have been too small to produce clear-cut results, and perhaps because of this there has been a tendency to give undue weight to epidemiological data, and even to base treatment directly on such evidence. Several different factors have often been manipulated simultaneously, making it difficult to tease out the contribution of individual components. Furthermore, the emphasis has been upon efficacy, with little attention to the tolerability, feasibility, expense, and even safety of the interventions. The outcome in short-term trials achieved with high levels of encouragement and support may not be attainable in routine long-term care. Interventions such as change of diet are often considered to be self-evidently beneficial and free of problems, but data will be discussed which shows such assumptions are not justified. These considerations may be particularly important in the elderly. They may, for example, be particularly prone to enhanced orthostatic responses to sodium restriction; they could find weight loss by calorie reduction difficult because of lower energy expenditure; or diet change may prove too expensive because of limited income.

   In this review we will concentrate on the non-pharmacological treatments outlined in Table 7.1. Where possible we will give most weight to controlled intervention trials in the elderly, but in many areas extrapolation from epidemiological evidence and from studies in younger subjects is needed. Wherever possible we will consider whether any effect is maintained in the long term; whether patients are likely to achieve the required changes outside the confines of a controlled trial; whether the size of any response justifies the expense or disruption to life; and whether the measures are safe and tolerable. Ideally we would present evidence that non-pharmacological treatment reduces strokes and heart attacks as is the case for drug treatment, but so far no study of non-pharmacological treatment has had the power to show this.

Table 7.1   Non-pharmacological interventions to lower blood pressure

Dietary changes	*Behavioural methods*
↓ Weight	↑ Physical activity
↓ Alcohol	
↓ Salt	Stress management
↓ Total fats	
	Biofeedback
↑ Potassium	
↑ Calcium	
↑ Polyunsaturated/saturated fat ratio	
↑ Magnesium	
Vegetarian diet	

WEIGHT REDUCTION

Numerous studies have shown a strong relationship between body weight and blood pressure, which is independent of possible confounding factors such as sodium intake and sex (Gordon and Kannel, 1976; Havlik *et al.*, 1983; Heyden and Schneider, 1990). This relationship is independent of measurement artefact related to arm circumference. Moreover, increases in weight over time are paralleled by rises in blood pressure (Tyroler *et al.*, 1975). In young adults the contribution of obesity to hypertension is important with as many as 30% of cases being attributable to obesity, and in young men the figure may be as high as 60% (MacMahon *et al.*, 1984). However, the contribution of body weight or obesity to hypertension may be less in older subjects. The prevalence of obesity increases throughout adult life but plateaus in the seventh decade and then may fall. Furthermore there is evidence from self-reported data that the association between increasing weight and elevated blood pressure weakens with age (Stamler *et al.*, 1978). An artefactual element in the relation between body weight and blood pressure is less likely in the elderly because older subjects lose skeletal muscle and thus have reduced arm circumference (Burch and Shewey, 1973).

The effect of weight loss on blood pressure is well established for young and middle-aged subjects. For example Reisin *et al.* (1978) reported that weight loss averaging about 9 kg was associated with falls in blood pressure of 19/18 mmHg in untreated patients and 30/21 mmHg in patients taking drug therapy, when compared with subjects with no change in body weight. These blood pressure changes could not be explained by the reduction in sodium intake often seen with calorie restriction. In another study (Ramsay *et al.*, 1978) there was a blood pressure fall of 2.5/1.5 mmHg for each kilogram of weight lost (Fig. 7.1). In an overview of eight intervention studies Andrews concluded that substantial weight loss reduced blood pressure by about 15% – an effect much greater than that of other non-pharmacological treatments, and similar to the response to a single antihypertensive drug (Andrews *et al.*, 1982). Despite the evidence that weight loss lowers blood pressure there is considerable scepticism both amongst doctors and the public at large as to the feasibility of losing weight and keeping it off. The evidence that there is for weight loss in hypertensive subjects would not support this view. Ramsay and colleagues (1978) examined the efficacy of three methods of helping hypertensive patients lose weight, all of which were suitable for primary or hospital care. The methods were doctor's advice, doctor's advice backed up by a written diet sheet, and referral to a dietician. The patients referred to the dietician achieved a significantly greater weight loss at 1 year (5.1 kg) but those given verbal or written advice still managed a useful reduction of 2.3 kg (Ramsay *et al.*, 1978). Interestingly a survey of compliance with weight reducing diets suggested that older females achieved a far greater weight reduction than

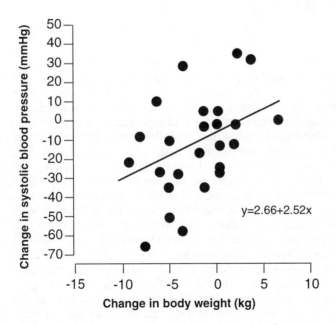

Fig. 7.1   Changes in blood pressure related to changes in body weight over 1 year in hypertensive patients. Figure adapted from Ramsay *et al.* (1978)

either older males or younger adults of either sex (Ramsay, 1985). Another controlled study including calorie restriction as one of its limbs demonstrated that a significant weight loss of about 5% body mass could be maintained for 4 years (Stamler *et al.*, 1987).

There is little evidence about the facility with which older subjects lose weight. As age increases there is a fall in muscle bulk and with this a fall in resting metabolic rate. The elderly have to eat far less to maintain a stable body weight and thus more severe restriction might be required to induce weight loss. Because of this it is not clear how evidence for younger subjects translates to hypertension in the elderly, especially as data for elderly subjects is sparse. In one controlled study (Applegate *et al.*, 1992) combined intervention by weight reduction, sodium restriction and increased exercise was examined over 6 months in elderly subjects. There was significant weight reduction of 1.8 kg, without any significant change in sodium excretion, and blood pressure fell by 4/5 mmHg. This was interpreted as showing that weight reduction lowered blood pressure in overweight elderly subjects with mild hypertension. However, this is confounded by the small fall in sodium excretion observed, even though it failed to achieve statistical significance. The study does demonstrate that some weight loss can be achieved and maintained for 6 months in elderly subjects, but the level of intervention was intense, involving as it did weekly sessions for the first 10 weeks (Applegate *et al.*, 1992).

In summary, the combination of strong epidemiological evidence, the intervention data for weight loss in younger subjects, and the small amount of data available in elderly subjects suggest that weight loss has a role to play in the management of high blood pressure in the elderly.

ALCOHOL

Regular alcohol consumption is positively associated with blood pressure in numerous cross-sectional population studies. One of the first of these, the Kaiser–Permanente study (Klatsky *et al.*, 1977), showed that subjects having three or more alcoholic drinks each day had significantly higher blood pressure than those who abstained or drank less than this amount. The effect of alcohol was independent of many potential confounding factors such as age, sex, race, smoking, coffee use, former heavy drinking, level of education, weight and dietary sodium. However in a later publication the same group highlighted a stronger association of blood pressure and alcohol with increasing age, and with male sex (Klatsky *et al.*, 1986). A separate cross-sectional study from Michigan showed the opposite suggesting that the blood pressure–alcohol relationship was more marked in younger adults and in women (Weissfeld *et al.*, 1988). Nevertheless, the authors predicted that men aged 60 or over who consumed >2 drinks per day had on average a systolic blood pressure 3.3 mmHg higher than those whose alcohol intake was lower. The equivalent difference for women aged over 60 years consuming >2 drinks per day was 10.4 mmHg (Weissfeld *et al.*, 1988).

It is difficult to judge how important a role alcohol may play in the aetiology of hypertension in the elderly. Across ages and sexes it has been estimated that 1% of a Western population will have high blood pressure due to alcohol, but in men this figure rises to 7% (Bulpitt *et al.*, 1987). In heavy-drinking men who consume more than 50 drinks each week the prevalence of hypertension rises further to 13%. In hypertensive men who drink heavily the raised blood pressure can be attributed directly to alcohol use in 33% (Bulpitt *et al.*, 1987). In older populations the frequency of regular drinkers falls dramatically in both sexes, yet the prevalence of hypertension increases (Weissfeld *et al.*, 1988). The likelihood of regular alcohol being the cause of hypertension will thus be much less in the elderly. Nevertheless alcohol may play a significant role in the aetiology of raised blood pressure in individual elderly subjects.

The epidemiological evidence of an association between alcohol and hypertension is supported by intervention studies, although these proved difficult. Saunders and colleagues (1981) studied regular drinkers with hypertension who were admitted to hospital. With withdrawal of alcohol blood pressure fell, only to rise again when alcohol was reintroduced. The best studies in both normotensive and hypertensive subjects are those of Puddey *et al.* (1985, 1987). Normotensive men were given either low or normal alcohol beer for 6 weeks in a randomised cross-over study (Puddey *et al.*, 1985). Systolic blood pressure rose by 1.1 mmHg for each 100 ml of alcohol consumed per week. In an identical study of treated hypertensive men who drank regularly, reducing the alcohol intake from 452 to 64 ml (57 to 8 units) per week caused a small fall in blood pressure averaging 5/3 mmHg. This was independent of any weight loss (Table 7.2) (Puddey *et al.*, 1987). The blood pressure fall was small, similar to that seen in normotensive men, probably because the patients were treated and had controlled blood pressures averaging 143/85 mmHg. The effect of alcohol moderation in untreated or poorly controlled hypertensives may be larger. However, in patients with blood pressure near the threshold for drug treatment, or when non-pharmacological intervention is used as an adjunct to drug treatment, a blood pressure fall of about 5/3 mmHg may be anticipated.

Little is known about the efficacy of advice on alcohol reduction in routine practice. One recent study (Maheswaran *et al.*, 1992) suggests that advice given in the hypertension clinic improved blood pressure control by an average of 5 mmHg diastolic, maintained for 8 weeks. Reported alcohol intake was halved from 60 to 30 units per week, and there was concomitant improvement in markers of liver damage, with a 21% reduction in gamma-glutamyl transferase (gamma-GT) (Maheswaran *et al.*, 1992). The effect of advice to reduce alcohol as a means of controlling blood pressure in elderly hypertensive subjects has not been formally studied. However, the strong epidemiological evidence, and the intervention data in middle-aged subjects, suggest that regular alcohol can be an important cause of hypertension. It should be sought and modified whatever the age of the patient.

DIETARY SODIUM

Many between-population studies have reported a relationship between the mean sodium intake, as estimated by 24-hour urinary sodium excretion, and the population blood pressure (Elliot, 1991). However, between-population studies may be seriously confounded by other factors, which could explain blood pressure differences. For example underdeveloped populations tend to be those with the lowest sodium intake. Within-population, cross-sectional studies have not shown a

Table 7.2 Effect of change in alcohol consumption on supine and standing blood pressure, weight, and gamma-glutamyl transferase in 40 moderate to heavy drinking men with stable, treated, essential hypertension

	Run-in (59 units/week)	Low alcohol (8 units/week)	Normal alcohol (57 units/week)	Difference low–high alcohol (−49 units/week)	P
Blood pressure:					
Supine (mmHg)	143/85	137/81	142/84	−5/−3	<0.001
Standing (mmHg)	137/89	128/83	134/86	−6/−3	<0.01
Weight* (kg)	82.2	81.5	82.4	−0.9	<0.001
Gamma-glutamyl transferase	52.7	37.6	50.8	−13.2	<0.001

*Effect of alcohol reduction on blood pressure independent from change in weight.
Adapted from Puddey *et al.* (1987).

clear relation of sodium intake to blood pressure, perhaps because of large within-subject variability in 24-hour urine excretion as compared to the small range of sodium intakes within populations. For Intersalt (Intersalt Cooperative Research Group, 1989), the across-population analysis was dominated by populations with particularly low sodium intakes, and when these were excluded there was no simple relation between sodium intake and blood pressure. However, there was a positive correlation between sodium intake and blood pressure in most populations, although it was not always statistically significant. When the regression coefficients were combined there was a highly significant but weak positive correlation between sodium intake and blood pressure (Intersalt Cooperative Research Group, 1989). Furthermore the increase in blood pressure with age was accentuated in those populations with a high sodium intake.

Evidence from intervention studies of sodium restriction is more convincing. In mildly hypertensive patients, MacGregor and colleagues (1982) used double-blind methodology, supplementing a low sodium diet with either slow sodium tablets or placebo to produce a difference in sodium intake of 80 mmol per day. There was a difference in mean blood pressure of 7 mmHg between the high and low sodium groups over a period of 4 weeks (MacGregor *et al.*, 1982). They subsequently confirmed the effect of sodium restriction with a sodium intake dose–response curve between 50–200 mmol per day (MacGregor *et al.*, 1989). Others could not reproduce these findings and this caused considerable debate at the time (Watt *et al.*, 1983). However, an overview of intervention trials confirmed efficacy, and also showed a strong relationship between the fall in blood pressure and the starting blood pressure (Grobbee and Hofman, 1986a). In the same overview age also had an important effect on antihypertensive response, with older subjects more responsive to the effects of sodium restriction. On average, 60-year-olds had a blood pressure fall with sodium restriction 2.5/3.0 mmHg larger than that of 30-year-olds (Grobbee and Hofman, 1986a). This was later confirmed by a single study (Australia National Health and Medical Research Council Dietary Salt Study Management Committee, 1989) in which 111 untreated hypertensive subjects were advised on a low sodium diet, and then randomised to placebo or to 80 mmol of slow sodium daily for 8 weeks. Sodium restriction reduced urinary sodium excretion by 71 mmol per 24 hours, and lowered blood pressure by 6/3 mmHg. The importance of starting blood pressure and age were confirmed, with older subjects again having the greater blood pressure fall. The increased response of older subjects to sodium restriction is not unexpected, as they tend to have low-renin, volume-dependent hypertension, and total body sodium correlates strongly with age in the hypertensive population (Beretta-Piccoli *et al.*, 1982).

Intervention studies in elderly hypertensive subjects have confirmed blood pressure reduction with sodium restriction. In a cross-over trial in patients with a mean age of 73 years, Fotherby and Potter (1993) attained a reduction in sodium intake of 80 mmol per 24 hours, and small falls in clinic and 24-hour blood pressures averaging 8/0 and 3/1 mmHg, respectively. Sodium restriction had no important effect on orthostatic blood pressure changes. Nestel and colleagues (1993) investigated the effects of sodium restriction, and of supplementing the diet with n-6 polyunsaturated fatty acids. Fatty acid loading had no effect on blood pressure, and the groups with and without dietary fat changes were combined to investigate the effect of sodium restriction. Women of mean age 65 years showed a significant fall in blood pressure, averaging 6/2 mmHg, and the size of the response was dependent on the starting blood pressure. The effect in men of mean age 66 years was very small, averaging only 0.8/0.5 mmHg, and was not statistically significant. In this study (Nestel *et al.*, 1993), men had a significantly higher sodium intake and higher blood pressures at the outset, and one might have anticipated larger falls in blood pressure when compared with women.

Much has been made of the potential benefit of reducing the population intake of sodium in order to lower blood pressure, but any effect on the blood pressure of individuals with normal or only mildly elevated blood pressure is likely to be very small. In those with moderate or severe hypertension, salt restriction will probably have a larger effect, but these patients are likely to need drug treatment anyway. Dietary sodium restriction appears to have an additive effect to drug treatment, at least with beta-blockers and angiotensin-converting enzyme inhibitors (Ertweman *et al.*, 1984; MacGregor *et al.*, 1987). The value of sodium restriction in practice will depend upon its tolerability and safety, and there is little information on this for elderly subjects. Combined non-pharmacological interventions in elderly subjects failed to achieve a significant fall in sodium excretion over 6 months (Applegate *et al.*, 1992), and the fall was much less than that seen in younger subjects after 4 years (Stamler *et al.*, 1987). This casts some doubt on the feasibility of such sodium restricted diets in older subjects.

In summary, while some studies suggest that the elderly are likely to have a more pronounced response to sodium restriction, this is not supported by intervention trials in elderly hypertensive patients. As evidence is lacking of a useful effect on blood pressure, and on feasibility and tolerability in the long term, sodium restriction has only a small role in the management of the elderly hypertensive patient.

OTHER CATIONS

Potassium

Epidemiological studies show a significant negative correlation between potassium intake as measured by 24-hour urinary potassium excretion and blood pressure (Langford, 1987). However, the association is weak, inconsistent, and possibly confounded by alcohol intake and social class (Beilin, 1988). Several randomised, controlled trials in which potassium intake was roughly doubled have shown a small blood pressure lowering effect. For example, Siani and colleagues (1987) reported significantly lower blood pressure with addition of 48 mmol potassium daily when compared with a control group. This difference reached a maximum of 14/11 mmHg after 15 weeks. However, not all trials have shown this, and to reconcile the findings Swales (1988) related responses to pre-intervention blood pressure as had been done for studies of sodium restriction. There was a clear relation between the blood pressure fall with potassium supplements and the starting blood pressure (Fig. 7.2). Patients who are already sodium restricted do not appear to have a further blood pressure response to potassium supplementation (Smith *et al.*, 1985) and it is possible that these two

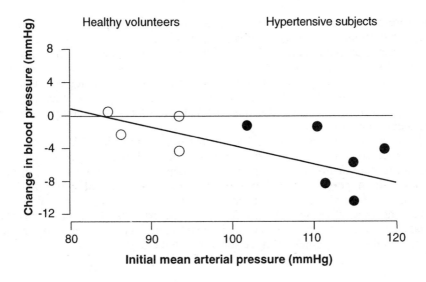

Fig. 7.2 Relationship between hypotensive response and initial blood pressure in studies examining the effect of potassium supplements on blood pressure. Data based on Swales (1988)

interventions work via a final common pathway, namely reduction in total body sodium. This hypothesis is supported by the natriuresis seen when patients receive potassium supplements (Zoccali *et al.*, 1985).

Fotherby and Potter (1992) investigated the effect of 4 weeks' treatment with potassium supplements in elderly patients with high blood pressure. Using a placebo-controlled, cross-over design they allocated elderly patients (mean age 75 years) to either potassium 60 mmol/day or placebo. Blood pressure responses were measured both by clinic readings and ambulatory blood pressure monitoring. The blood pressure response to potassium was 10/6 mmHg for clinic readings and 5/2 mmHg for average daytime readings by ambulatory monitoring. There was no important orthostatic blood pressure fall with potassium supplements. The large fall in clinic blood pressure was probably due to the high initial pressure, of 181/97 mmHg, consistent with the relationship reported by Swales (1988) (Fig. 7.2). Potassium supplements will occasionally cause dangerous hyperkalaemia, and the elderly are more likely to be susceptible to this due to their limited renal functional reserve.

Calcium

The role of calcium in the control of blood pressure is much less clear than that of sodium or potassium. Data from nutritional surveys imply that there may be an inverse correlation between calcium in the diet and blood pressure. However, this is not a universal finding and some of the surveys have been criticised for the methods used to assess calcium intake (Kaplan and Meese, 1986; McCarron and Morris, 1985a; Resnick, 1987). Studies relating plasma calcium to blood pressure do not give a uniform picture. The larger studies generally show a positive correlation, making it unlikely that calcium deficiency is a major cause of hypertension (Kaplan and Meese, 1986). In a cross-sectional study of elderly women (Simon et al., 1992) there was a weak but statistically significant correlation between dietary calcium, assessed from a food frequency questionnaire, and blood pressure. However, age, body-mass index, alcohol consumption and attained level of education all had a far greater influence on blood pressure than did dietary calcium.

Intravenous calcium elevates blood pressure acutely, but the effects of oral supplementation are variable, with different studies showing either a small fall in blood pressure or no change. The most frequent finding is a small fall in blood pressure in hypertensive patients, of the order of 2–3 mmHg (Grobbee and Hofman, 1986b; McCarron and Morris, 1985b), and no change in the blood pressure of normotensive subjects (McCarron and Morris, 1985b). Considering these small responses it is unlikely that calcium supplementation has an important role to play in the management of hypertension in the elderly.

Magnesium

Cross-sectional surveys do not suggest a relationship between dietary magnesium intake and blood pressure (Harlan et al., 1984). Studies relating serum magnesium to blood pressure show all possible outcomes, with high serum magnesium predicting high blood pressure or low blood pressure (Albert et al., 1958; Petersen et al., 1977; Walker and Walker, 1936). Early studies of magnesium supplementation in patients on diuretic treatment for hypertension (Dyckner and Wester, 1983; Reyes et al., 1984) suggested that magnesium lowered blood pressure, but this was refuted by a larger controlled study (Henderson et al., 1986). In untreated patients magnesium had no effect on blood pressure (Cappuccio et al., 1985), but a recent study in middle-aged and elderly women (Witteman et al., 1994) showed a blood pressure fall with magnesium supplements averaging 3/3 mmHg at 6 months. The inconsistent findings in epidemiological and intervention studies, and the very small effect on blood pressure even in positive studies, indicate that magnesium supplements should not figure in the routine management of hypertension.

Combined dietary supplements

Many studies investigating the effects of modifying dietary intake of cations have attempted to alter them in combination. Do interventions which proved disappointing when used alone produce a worthwhile blood pressure fall in combination? Geleijnse and his colleagues (1994) investigated the role of potassium and magnesium supplements in patients taking a low sodium diet in 100 elderly hypertensive subjects. They were randomised to receive either a high potassium, high magnesium salt to use in cooking and at the table, or to use ordinary salt for cooking and at the table, and were followed for 24 weeks. During the final 16 weeks of the study blood pressure was 8/3 mmHg lower in the intervention than the control group, and there were no differences in reported adverse effects (Geleijnse *et al.*, 1994). However, the power of the study to detect possible adverse events was low. This study shows potential benefit from non-pharmacological treatment, but it would be difficult to implement such intervention widely. The subjects were provided with special foodstuffs free of charge and were contacted each month to encourage compliance. The response to combined modification of dietary salts seems greater than that to individual changes in salts, but the effect on blood pressure remains small compared to those with weight loss or alcohol reduction.

Other diets

Vegetarian diet

There is a body of evidence from blood pressure surveys that vegetarian diets are associated with lower blood pressure. In a comparison of two religious groups which avoided alcohol, tobacco and caffeine, blood pressure was lower in lacto ovo vegetarians than meat eaters, and this was independent of body weight, age and sex (Rouse *et al.*, 1983a). This effect may persist into old age (Melby *et al.*, 1993). However the differences between dietary groups may be explained by variations in body mass. In randomised controlled trials in middle-aged subjects, changing from an omnivorous diet to a vegetarian diet lowers blood pressure by about 6/3 mmHg in normotensive subjects (Rouse *et al.*, 1983b), and by 4 mmHg systolic in hypertensive subjects (Margetts *et al.*, 1986), independent of any fall in body weight or sodium intake. It is not clear which components of omnivorous and vegetarian diets are responsible for the differences in blood pressure. It is doubtful whether subjects will forgo animal products in the diet for reasons of health.

Dietary fats

There is evidence from intervention studies that changing the type of dietary fat may reduce blood pressure, although more attention has been paid to changes in other cardiovascular risk factors such as hyperlipidaemia. In one controlled trial, reducing total fat to 25% of calorie intake and increasing the polyunsaturated to saturated fat ratio to one, a fairly rigorous diet, caused a significant fall in blood pressure of 7/3 mmHg at 6 weeks (Puska *et al.*, 1983). Linoleic acid supplements alone do not alter blood pressure, but significant falls in blood pressure are reported with increases in marine polyunsaturated fats (Knapp and Fitzgerald, 1989). One study in elderly subjects showed no effect of marine oils alone on blood pressure, but there was a small blood pressure fall when combined with a low sodium diet (Cobiac *et al.*, 1992). The doses of fish oil required to lower blood pressure appear high when compared to those shown to reduce coronary death after myocardial infarction (Burr *et al.*, 1989), and they could not be achieved by increasing the amount of fish in the diet. Fish oils would have to be taken in pharmacological doses in capsule form, and their efficacy and safety for long-term treatment need rigorous evaluation.

Exercise and other behavioural methods

Some epidemiological studies suggest a beneficial effect of exercise on blood pressure but others such as Framingham (Kannel, 1980) show no relationship. An overview suggests that there may be a weak inverse relationship between exercise and blood pressure after correcting for age and weight (Fagard, 1985). Intervention studies on the effect of exercise have not added greatly to our knowledge. They have generally been poorly designed, and it is impossible to blind such studies. Possible confounding factors include changes in body weight and diet with increasing exercise. An overview of the better controlled studies (Fagard *et al.*, 1990) suggests an average antihypertensive response to exercise training of 4/4 mmHg in normotensive subjects, and 11/6 mmHg in those with hypertension. The fall in blood pressure was again strongly related to initial blood pressure, but not to age. There is debate about the extent of training required to achieve these benefits. Braith and colleagues (1994) investigated the effect of moderate- and high-intensity exercise on blood pressure in elderly normotensive subjects aged 60 to 79 years. After a 3-week baseline period the intervention groups trained up to 70% of predicted maximum heart rate in the moderate group, and to 80–85% in the high intensity group. Exercise was performed three times each week and maintained for 6 months. Blood pressure responses were similar in both exercise groups, averaging 8/11 mmHg when compared with a control group. Surprisingly there was no change in body weight, but skinfold thickness decreased, suggesting that loss of body fat was balanced by an increase in muscle bulk. Elderly subjects do not generally take much exercise, and there are other potential benefits on work capacity and even osteoporosis. The role of acceptable exercise in elderly hypertensive patients deserves study.

The antihypertensive effects of biofeedback and relaxation have been studied extensively, but unfortunately many of the studies have been poorly designed (Swales, 1988). The outcome in 24 studies of behavioural treatment of hypertension has been reviewed (Anonymous, 1989). There was no significant difference in blood pressure between treatment and control groups in 11 studies, and significant falls of blood pressure in 'treated' patients in 13. Few studies have examined these techniques in the longer term, they are time-consuming, and different therapists may obtain different results with similar programmes. These techniques have a certain attraction, but their suitability for general use has not been proven either in middle-aged or elderly patients.

Non-pharmacological measures in combination

In ordinary practice the non-pharmacological treatments discussed above are not used in isolation, but in combination. Long-term controlled trials of non-pharmacological regimens lasting 1–4 years have been performed in middle-aged hypertensive patients, and the results raise points of considerable importance. The principal components of the regimens studied were weight, salt and alcohol reduction. One major finding was that these measures could be successfully implemented and maintained over long periods (Berglund *et al.*, 1989; Stamler *et al.*, 1987). The interventions also lowered blood pressure, and had a significant 'treatment-sparing' effect when compared with control groups not given non-pharmacological advice (Stamler *et al.*, 1987). Expressed simply, a proportion of hypertensive subjects given comprehensive non-pharmacological advice can avoid antihypertensive drugs. This can be interpreted as showing that non-pharmacological treatments were advantageous, but careful analysis suggests that this may not be the case, as discussed below.

Non-pharmacological management versus drug therapy

The results of two trials comparing non-pharmacological intervention and drug treatment reveal the true benefits and costs of avoiding drug therapy. The first, reported by Berglund *et al.* (1989), was a direct comparison of non-pharmacological therapy versus antihypertensive drug treatment over 1 year in obese men aged 40–69 with untreated hypertension (90–104 mmHg diastolic). The dietary intervention included weight reduction, moderate salt restriction, and alcohol reduction, in addition to increases in dietary potassium and in the ratio of polyunsaturated to saturated fats. In the group treated with antihypertensive drugs a stepped-care approach was followed, with atenolol as first-line treatment. The findings after 1 year were:

- significant net reductions in body weight of 8.5 kg and sodium excretion of 32 mmol daily in the diet group. Reported alcohol intake and urine potassium excretion did not differ between the groups;
- those treated by diet had significantly higher blood pressure than those treated by drugs after 1 year, with mean values 147/92 mmHg and 140/86 mmHg respectively. Diastolic blood pressure was 90 mmHg or lower in 29% of patients treated by diet, compared with 73% of those treated by drugs;
- diet-treated patients had lower concentrations of total cholesterol, LDL cholesterol and triglycerides, and higher levels of HDL cholesterol.

The blood pressure response to non-pharmacological treatment was disappointing, considering particularly the substantial weight loss. Those given drug therapy had a significant blood pressure 'advantage' averaging 7/6 mmHg, and a 'disadvantage' as regards lipid changes of 0.37 mmol/L in total cholesterol. In the absence of long-term outcome data with these regimens we have to fall back on epidemiological and clinical trial data (Collins *et al.*, 1990; MacMahon *et al.*, 1990) to predict what such differences might mean. A diastolic blood pressure difference averaging 6 mmHg might translate to a 40% increase in stroke risk and a 20–25% increase in coronary risk in those given non-pharmacological treatment only. This would far outweigh any difference in coronary risk related to the lower serum cholesterol concentration. When compared head-to-head, anti-hypertensive drug treatment appears markedly superior to non-pharmacological management.

A straight comparison of these forms of treatment is not directly relevant to ordinary practice because non-pharmacological therapy is recommended as an adjunct to drug treatment, not an alternative. The Hypertension Control Program (Stamler *et al.*, 1987) examined precisely this strategy over a 4-year period. Men and women aged on average 56 years, with mild hypertension controlled by anti-hypertensive drugs, and who were slightly overweight, were randomly allocated to one of three groups. They would continue drug therapy without dietary intervention; withdrawal off drug therapy plus dietary intervention; or withdrawal off drug therapy with no dietary intervention. The non-pharmacological interventions included weight reduction, moderate salt restriction, and alcohol reduction where appropriate. Bearing in mind that all patients were treated and normotensive at entry, the principle endpoint was a rise in blood pressure during follow-up to a diastolic pressure consistently above 90 mmHg, requiring reinstitution of antihypertensive drugs. The principle findings at the end of the trial were:

- dietary intervention achieved significant net reductions in body weight averaging 3.8 kg, and sodium excretion averaging 53 mmol/L, and a non-significant reduction in reported alcohol use.
- after 4 years 39% of those given dietary advice remained normotensive and off drug therapy.
- those randomised to dietary advice, whether or not they had to restart drug therapy, had significantly higher blood pressure after 4 years, by a mean of 11/4 mmHg.
- those given dietary advice who stayed off drug therapy had lower levels of serum cholesterol and fasting glucose than those who continued on drug therapy.

There was therefore an important 'treatment-sparing' effect of non-pharmacological treatment, with almost 40% of patients able to avoid drugs for 4 years. The disadvantage was of course the difference between the groups in blood pressure at the end of the study. The group who had non-pharmacological advice, with addition of drug therapy as an adjunct when needed, had higher blood pressure by an average of 11/4 mmHg. By extrapolation from epidemiological and intervention trial data (Collins *et al.*, 1990; MacMahon *et al.*, 1990) those given non-pharmacological advice may have avoided drug therapy at the expense of a substantially increased risk of cardiovascular complications. Intensive advice on non-pharmacological measures before starting drug therapy resulted in significantly inferior blood pressure control in the whole population of patients.

Sub-optimal blood pressure control is not the only possible drawback of non-pharmacological intervention. The TAIM study (Wassertheil-Smoller *et al.*, 1991) examined two non-pharmacological treatments and two drug treatments for hypertension in factorial design. The diets studied were a normal diet; a low sodium and high potassium; and a calorie restricted diet; and the drugs were placebo, atenolol and low-dose chlorthalidone. The main endpoints were quality of life scores and sexual function. The weight reducing diet achieved a reduction in weight averaging 4.7 kg at 6 months, lowered blood pressure when combined with placebo, and enhanced the blood pressure responses to chlorthalidone and to atenolol. Additionally, patients who were allocated to weight reduction reported significant reductions in physical and sexual problems, and an increase in satisfaction with physical health. However, patients allocated to the low sodium and high potassium diet reported no change in physical health but were more likely to suffer fatigue. Patients on this diet plus drug therapy reported an increase in sleep disturbance. These differences between the two non-pharmacological interventions highlight the important point that non-pharmacological treatments should not be embraced uncritically because they are simple and effective. Their effect on quality of life and their potential to cause harm need to be examined just as carefully as have those of antihypertensive drugs.

DISCUSSION

Non-pharmacological interventions appear at least as effective in controlling blood pressure in elderly subjects as they are in middle age. Weight reduction and salt restriction have been shown to lower blood pressure in controlled trials in the elderly. There are no direct data for alcohol reduction specific to older hypertensives, but extrapolation from trials in younger patients appears to be justified. The precise role of these non-pharmacological interventions depends critically on their tolerability and efficacy when compared with drug treatment. We have reservations about the use of non-pharmacological measures in an attempt to avoid drug therapy. The outcome of the Hypertension Control Program (Stamler *et al.*, 1987) suggests that vigorous implementation of non-pharmacological treatment may result in sub-optimal blood pressure control and leave patients at an increased risk of cardiovascular complications when compared with those treated by drugs. Zealous implementation of non-pharmacological treatment may have been appropriate when the only drugs available for hypertension were sympathetic blockers, centrally acting drugs, high dosage of thiazides and non-selective beta-blockers. Such treatment was poorly tolerated and complex for both doctor and patient. It was treatment worth avoiding at almost any cost. However, recent large studies (Materson *et al.*, 1993; Treatment of Mild Hypertension Research Group, 1991; Wassertheil-Smoller *et al.*, 1991), some including sophisticated measures of quality of life indicate that low-dose thiazide, selective beta-blockers, and newer drugs such as angiotensin-converting enzyme inhibitors and calcium antagonists are remarkably well-tolerated. Considering also the simplicity of modern treatment regimens, and the substantial reduction in cardiovascular complications attained (Collins *et al.*, 1990), particularly in the elderly (MRC Working Party, 1992; SHEP Cooperative Research Group, 1991), strenuous efforts to avoid such treatment through advice on non-pharmacological measures should perhaps be tempered.

CONCLUSIONS

Weight reduction, moderate salt restriction and alcohol reduction undoubtedly lower blood pressure, and are likely to be at least as effective in the elderly as in younger hypertensives. However, intensive advice on non-pharmacological measures may leave patients at some disadvantage. The cost of avoiding anti-hypertensive drug therapy may be sub-optimal blood pressure control and prevention of the cardiovascular complications of hypertension. Elderly patients with hypertension established by repeated measurements over an adequate period of observation should have their blood pressure lowered below 160 mmHg systolic and 90 mmHg diastolic. Substantial benefits in morbidity and mortality are likely to be attained only if treatment achieves a substantial blood pressure fall. Intervention trials in elderly hypertensive subjects, which have been conspicuously successful in preventing cardiovascular complications at remarkably little cost as regards adverse effects, have aimed for reductions in systolic blood pressure of 20–30 mmHg. Blood pressure falls of this magnitude are unlikely to be achieved by non-pharmacological treatment alone.

REFERENCES

Albert DG, Morita Y, Iseri LT 1958. Serum magnesium and plasma sodium levels in essential vascular hypertension. *Circulation* **17**, 1761–4.

Andrews G, MacMahon SW, Austin A, Byrne DG 1982. Hypertension: comparison of drug and non drug treatments. *British Medical Journal* **284**, 1523–6.

Anonymous 1989. Relaxation therapy for hypertensive patients. *Drug and Therapeutics Bulletin* **27**, 77–9.

Applegate WB, Miller ST, Elam JT *et al.* 1992. Nonpharmacologic intervention to reduce blood pressure in older patients with mild hypertension. *Archives of Internal Medicine* **152**, 1162–6.

Australia National Health and Medical Research Council Dietary Salt Study Management Committee 1989. Fall in blood pressure with moderate reduction in dietary salt intake in mild hypertension. *Lancet* **i**, 399–402.

Beilin LJ 1988. Non-pharmacological control of blood pressure. *Clinical and Experimental Pharmacology and Physiology* **15**, 215–23.

Beretta-Piccoli C, Davies DL, Boddy K *et al.* 1982. Relation of arterial pressure with body sodium, body potassium and plasma potassium in essential hypertension. *Clinical Science* **63**, 257–70.

Berglund A, Andersson OK, Berglund G, Fagerberg B 1989. Antihypertensive effect of diet compared with drug treatment in obese men with mild hypertension. *British Medical Journal* **299**, 480–5.

Braith RW, Pollock ML, Lowenthal DT, Graves JE, Leimacher MC 1994. Moderate and high intensity exercise lowers blood pressure in normotensive subjects 60 to 79 years of age. *American Journal of Cardiology* **73**, 1124–8.

Bulpitt CJ, Shipley MJ, Semmence A 1987. The contribution of a moderate intake of alcohol to the presence of hypertension. *Journal of Hypertension* **5**, 85–91.

Burch GE, Shewey L 1973. Sphygmomanometric cuff size and blood pressure recordings. *Journal of the American Medical Association* **225**, 1215–18.

Burr ML, Fehily AM, Gilbert JF *et al.* 1989. Effects of changes in fat, fish and fibre intakes on death and myocardial reinfarction: diet and reinfarction trial (DART). *Lancet* **ii**, 757–61.

Cappuccio FP, Markandu MD, Benyon GW, Shore AC, Sampson B, MacGregor GA 1985. Lack of effect of oral magnesium: a double blind study. *British Medical Journal* **291**, 235–8.

Cobiac L, Nestel PJ, Wing LMH, Howe PRC 1992. A low sodium diet supplemented with fish oil lowers blood pressure in the elderly. *Journal of Hypertension* **10**, 87–92.

Collins R, Peto R, MacMahon S *et al.* 1990. Blood pressure, stroke and coronary heart disease. II Short term reductions in blood pressure: overview of randomised drug trials in their epidemiological context. *Lancet* **335**, 827–38.

Dyckner T, Wester PO 1983. Effects of magnesium on blood pressure. *British Medical Journal* **286**, 1847–9.

Elliot P 1991. Observational studies of salt and blood pressure. *Hypertension* **17**(Suppl. 1), 13–18.

Ertweman TM, Naglekerke N, Lubsen J, Koster M, Dunning AJ 1984. Beta blockade, diuretics and salt restriction for the management of hypertension: a randomised double blind trial. *British Medical Journal* **289**, 406–9.

Fagard R 1985. Habitual physical activity, training and blood pressure in normo- and hypertension. *International Journal of Sports Medicine* **6**, 57–67.

Fagard R, Bielin E, Hespel P *et al.* 1990. Physical exercise in hypertension. In Laragh JH, Brenner BM (eds) *Hypertension, pathophysiology, diagnosis and management.* New York: Raven, 1985–98.

Fotherby MD, Potter JF 1992. Potassium supplementation reduces clinic and ambulatory blood pressure in elderly hypertensive patients. *Journal of Hypertension* **10**, 1403–8.

Fotherby MD, Potter JF 1993. Effects of moderate sodium restriction on clinic and twenty-four hour ambulatory blood pressure in elderly hypertensive subjects. *Journal of Hypertension* **11**, 657–63.

Geleijnse JM, Witteman JCM, Bak AAA, den Breeijen JH, Grobbee DE 1994. Reduction in blood pressure with a low sodium, high potassium, high magnesium salt in older subjects with mild to moderate hypertension. *British Medical Journal* **309**, 436–40.

Gordon T, Kannel WB 1976. Obesity and cardiovascular diseases: the Framingham study. *Clinical Endocrinology and Metabolism* **5**, 367–75.

Grobbee DE, Hofman A 1986a. Does sodium restriction lower blood pressure? *British Medical Journal* **293**, 27–9.

Grobbee DE, Hofman A 1986b. Effect of calcium supplementation on diastolic blood pressure in young people with mild hypertension. *Lancet* **ii**, 703–6.

Harlan WR, Hull LA, Schmouder RL, Landis JR, Thompson FE, Larkin FA 1984. Blood pressure and nutrition in adults: the national Health and Nutrition Examination Survey. *American Journal of Epidemiology* **120**, 17–18.

Havlik RJ, Hubert HB, Fabsitz RR, Feinleib M 1983. Weight and hypertension. *Annals of Internal Medicine* **98**, 855–9.

Henderson DG, Scherys J, Schott T 1986. Effect of magnesium supplementation on blood pressure and electrolyte concentrations in hypertensive patients receiving long-term diuretic treatment. *British Medical Journal* **293**, 664–5.

Heyden S, Schneider KA 1990. Obesity and hypertension: epidemiological aspects of the relationship. *Journal of Human Hypertension* **4**, 431–5.

Intersalt Cooperative Research Group 1989. The Intersalt study. *Journal of Human Hypertension* **3**, 279–320.

Kannel WB 1980. Host and environmental determinants of hypertension: perspective from the Framingham study. In Kestelfoot H, Joosens J (eds) *Epidemiology of arterial blood pressure.* The Hague: Martinus Nijhoff, 265–78.

Kaplan NM, Meese RB 1986. The calcium deficiency hypothesis of hypertension: a critique. *Annals of Internal Medicine* **105**, 947–55.

Klatsky AL, Freidman DG, Armstrong MA 1986. The relationships between alcoholic beverage use and other traits to blood pressure: a new Kaiser–Permanente study. *Circulation* **73**, 628–36.

Klatsky AL, Freidman DG, Siegelaub AB, Gerard MJ 1977. Alcohol consumption and blood pressure: Kaiser–Permanente multiphasic health examination data. *New England Journal of Medicine* **296**, 1194–200.

Knapp HR, Fitzgerald GA 1989. The antihypertensive effects of fish oil: a controlled study of polyunsaturated fatty acid supplements in essential hypertension. *New England Journal of Medicine* **320**, 1037–43.

Langford HG 1987. Potassium and its role in the etiology and therapy of hypertension. In Blaufox MD, Langford HG (eds) *Bibliotheca cardiologica – non-pharmacologic therapy of hypertension.* Basel: Karger, Vol. 41, 57–68.

MacGregor GA, Markandu ND, Best FE *et al.* 1982. Double-blind randomised crossover trial of moderate sodium restriction in essential hypertension. *Lancet* **i**, 351–5.

MacGregor GA, Markandu ND, Sagnella GA, Singer DRJ, Cappuccio FP 1989. Double-blind study of three intakes and long-term effects of sodium restriction in essential hypertension. *Lancet* **ii**, 1244–7.

MacGregor GA, Markandu ND, Singer DRJ, Cappuccio FP, Shore AC, Sagnella GA 1987.

146 *Non-pharmacological treatment*

Moderate sodium restriction with angiotensin converting enzyme inhibitor in essential hypertension: a double blind study. *British Medical Journal* **294**, 531–4.

MacMahon SW, Blacket RB, Macdonald GJ, Hall W 1984. Obesity, alcohol consumption and blood pressure in Australian men and women. The National Heart Foundation of Australia risk factor prevalence study. *Journal of Hypertension* **2**, 85–91.

MacMahon S, Peto R, Cutler J *et al.* 1990. Blood pressure, stroke and coronary heart disease. Part 1, prolonged differences in blood pressure: prospective observational studies corrected for the regression dilution bias. *Lancet* **335**, 765–74.

Maheswaran R, Beevers M, Beevers DG 1992. Effectiveness of advice to reduce alcohol consumption in hypertensive patients. *Hypertension* **19**, 79–84.

Margetts BM, Beilin LJ, Vandongen R, Armstrong BK 1986. Vegetarian diet in mild hypertension: a randomised controlled trial. *British Medical Journal* **293**, 1468–71.

Materson BJ, Reda DJ, Cushman WC *et al.* for the Department of Veterans Affairs Cooperative Study Group on Antihypertensive Agents 1993. Single-drug therapy for hypertension in men. A comparison of six antihypertensive agents with placebo. *New England Journal of Medicine* **328**, 914–21.

McCarron DA, Morris CD 1985a. Calcium and hypertension: evidence for a protective action of the cation. In Horan MJ (ed.) *NIH workshop on nutrition and hypertension: Proceedings from a symposium.* Bethesda Maryland, Biomedical Information Corporation, 167–86.

McCarron DA, Morris C 1985b. Blood pressure response to oral calcium in persons with mild to moderate hypertension: A randomized, double-blind, placebo-controlled, crossover trial. *Annals of Internal Medicine* **103**, 825–31.

Melby CL, Goldflies DG, Toohey ML 1993. Blood pressure differences in older Black and White long-term vegetarians and nonvegetarians. *Journal of the American College of Nutrition* **12**, 262–9.

MRC Working Party 1992. Medical Research Council trials of treatment of hypertension in older adults: principal results. *British Medical Journal* **304**, 405–12.

Nestel PJ, Clifton PM, Noakes M, MacArthur R, Howe PR 1993. Enhanced blood pressure response to dietary salt in elderly women, especially those with small waist–hip ratio. *Journal of Hypertension* **11**, 1387–94.

Petersen E, Schroll M, Christiansen C, Transbel I 1977. Serum and erythrocyte magnesium in normal elderly Danish people: relationship to blood pressure and serum lipids. *Acta Medica Scandinavia* **201**, 31–4.

Puddey IB, Beilin LJ, Vandongen R 1987. Regular alcohol use raises blood pressure in treated hypertensive subjects. *Lancet* **i**, 647–51.

Puddey IB, Beilin LJ, Vandongen R, Rouse IL, Rogers P 1985. Evidence for a direct effect of alcohol consumption on blood pressure in normotensive men: A randomised controlled trial. *Hypertension* **7**, 707–13.

Puska P, Iacono JM, Nissenen A *et al.* 1983. Controlled, randomised trial of the effect of dietary fat on blood pressure. *Lancet* **ii**, 1–5.

Ramsay LE 1985. Compliance with weight reduction in hypertensive patients. *Journal of Hypertension* **3**(Suppl. 1), 81–5.

Ramsay LE, Ramsay MH, Hettiarachchi J, Davies DL, Winchester J 1978. Weight reduction in a blood pressure clinic. *British Medical Journal* **ii**, 244–5.

Reisin E, Abel R, Modan M, Silverberg DS, Eliahou HE, Modan B 1978. Effect of weight loss without salt restriction on the reduction of blood pressure in overweight hypertensive patients. *New England Journal of Medicine* **298**, 1–6.

Resnick LM 1987. Dietary calcium and hypertension. *Journal of Nutrition* **117**, 1806–8.

Reyes AJ, Leary WP, Acosta-Barrios TN, Davis WH 1984. Magnesium supplementation in hypertension treated with hydrochlorothiazide. *Current Therapeutic Research* **36**, 332–40.

Rouse IL, Armstrong BK, Beilin LJ 1983a. The relationship of blood pressure to diet and lifestyle in two religious populations. *Journal of Hypertension* **1**, 65–71.

Rouse IL, Beilin LJ, Armstrong BK, Vandongen R 1983b. Blood pressure lowering effect of a vegetarian diet: controlled trial in normotensive subjects. *Lancet* **i**, 5–10.

Saunders JB, Beevers DG, Paton A 1981. 'Alcohol-induced' hypertension. *Lancet* **ii**, 653–6.

SHEP Cooperative Research Group 1991. Prevention of stroke by antihypertensive drug treatment in older persons with isolated systolic hypertension. Final results of the Systolic Hypertension in the Elderly Program (SHEP). *Journal of the American Medical Association* **265**, 3255–64.

Siani A, Strazzullo P, Russo L *et al.* 1987. Controlled trial of long term oral potassium supplements in patients with mild hypertension. *British Medical Journal* **294**, 1453–6.

Simon JA, Browner WS, Tao JL, Hulley SB 1992. Calcium intake and blood pressure in elderly women. *American Journal of Epidemiology* **136**, 1241–7.

Smith SJ, Markandu ND, Sagnella GA, MacGregor GA 1985. Moderate potassium chloride supplementation in essential hypertension: is it additive to moderate sodium restriction? *British Medical Journal* **291**, 110–13.

Stamler R, Stamler J, Grimm R *et al.* 1987. Nutritional therapy for high blood pressure: final report of a four year randomized controlled trial – the Hypertension Control Program. *Journal of the American Medical Association* **257**, 1484–91.

Stamler R, Stamler J, Reidlinger WF, Algera G, Robertes RH 1978. Weight and blood pressure. Findings in hypertension screening of one million Americans. *Journal of the American Medical Association* **240**, 1607–10.

Swales JD 1988. Non-pharmacological antihypertensive therapy. *European Heart Journal* **9**(Suppl. G), 45–52.

Treatment of Mild Hypertension Research Group 1991. The treatment of mild hypertension study. A randomized placebo-controlled trial of a nutritional–hygienic regimen along with various drug monotherapies. *Archives of Internal Medicine* **151**, 1413–23.

Tyroler HA, Heydon S, Hames CG 1975. Weight and hypertension: Evans County studies of Blacks and Whites. In Paul O (ed.) *Epidemiology and control of hypertension*. New York: Stratton Intercontinental, 177–204.

Walker BS, Walker EW 1936. Normal magnesium metabolism and its significant disturbances. *Journal of Laboratory and Clinical Medicine* **21**, 713–20.

Wassertheil-Smoller S, Blaufox MD, Oberman A *et al.*, for the TAIM Research Group 1991. Effect of antihypertensives on sexual function and quality of life: the TAIM study. *Annals of Internal Medicine* **114**, 613–20.

Watt GCM, Edwards C, Hart JT, Hart M, Walton P, Foy CJW 1983. Dietary sodium restriction for mild hypertension in general practice. *British Medical Journal* **286**, 432–6.

Weissfeld JL, Johnson EH, Brock BM, Hawthorne VM 1988. Sex and age interactions in the association between alcohol and blood pressure. *American Journal of Epidemiology* **128**, 559–69.

Whelton PK, Adams Campbel II, Appel LJ *et al.* 1993. National high blood pressure education program working group report on primary prevention of hypertension. *Archives of Internal Medicine* **153**, 186–208.

Witteman JCM, Grobbee DE, Derkx FHM, Bouillon R, de Bruijn AM, Hofman A 1994. Reduction of blood pressure with oral magnesium supplementation in women with mild to moderate hypertension. *American Journal of Clinical Nutrition* **60**, 129–35.

Zoccali C, Cumming AMM, Hutcheson MJ, Barnett P, Semple PF 1985. Effect of potassium on sodium balance, renin, noradrenaline and arterial pressure. *Journal of Hypertension* **3**, 67–72.

CHAPTER 8

Cost-effectiveness of treating hypertension in the older adult

DOUGLAS COYLE

INTRODUCTION

In recent years there has been increasing attention on both the benefits and costs of new technologies. This is a direct result of increasing financial pressures on health care systems throughout the world. New technologies have increased the ability to improve health status, but at an increasing cost. Improvements in treatment as well as in diet and environment have led to an increasingly elderly population, with further resultant pressures on health care budgets.

Individual governments are putting pressure on decision-makers to control health care expenditure. This has led to both incentives for decision-makers to consider whether resources allocated to health technologies are allocated appropriately and formal requirements that technologies are proven to be cost-effective (Commonwealth of Australia, 1992; Ontario Ministry of Health, 1994). Changes to the systems of financing pharmaceutical expenditure have been one of the major methods by which governments have controlled overall health care expenditure. This has manifested itself in various ways. In certain countries, expenditure on pharmaceuticals has been controlled by the use of patient co-payments. In others, concern has focused on the cost-effectiveness of pharmaceuticals and has led to requirements for pharmaceutical companies to demonstrate the effectiveness and cost-effectiveness of new products before they are financed.

As a result, there is an increasing role for the assessment of new health technologies and specifically the economic evaluation of health technologies. This is reflected by the large rise in the number of economic evaluations of health care interventions in Europe. A recent review of economic evaluations of health care found only 33 European studies published between 1978 and 1982, while 114 studies were published between 1988 and 1992 (Backhouse *et al.*, 1992).

Given the concern for controlling pharmaceutical expenditure, the increasing number of innovatory products to treat disease and the increasing proportion of the population which is elderly, concern over the costs of treating hypertension has been evident. Various papers have included discussions of the relevance of cost-effectiveness in the treatment of hypertension (Robertson, 1989; Shaw, 1993; Whitcomb and Byyny, 1990). However, no definitive study of the cost-effectiveness of treatment for the elderly has been conducted. This chapter addresses the methods of establishing the cost-effectiveness of various alternative treatments for hypertension in the elderly.

The following section outlines the methods for conducting an economic evaluation of antihypertensive therapy (both pharmaceutical and non-pharmaceutical). The second section provides estimates of the current cost of treating hypertension in the elderly in the UK and the costs of treating those conditions that may be preventable through treatment (cerebrovascular and coronary heart disease). The third section provides a review of the available evidence of the cost-effectiveness of the alternatives available. Finally, the last section provides a discussion of what we do and do not know about the cost-effectiveness of treatments for hypertension in the elderly and what additional research is still required.

METHODS FOR ESTABLISHING THE COST-EFFECTIVENESS OF TREATMENTS

What is economic evaluation?

Economic evaluation provides an analytical framework for assessing both the costs and benefits of health technologies in a systematic manner (Drummond *et al.*, 1987). By adopting such a framework, technologies can be compared and those technologies that can be deemed to be of 'value for money' (cost-effective) can be identified. This section summarises the forms of analysis available and the methodological principles which studies should adhere to, and provides a model from which the cost-effectiveness of alternative treatments for hypertension in the elderly can be assessed.

Forms of analysis

In economic evaluation the method of measuring the benefit of technology varies according to the form of analysis conducted. There are four main forms of analyses which are employed (Table 8.1).

Table 8.1   Types of economic evaluation

	Cost measurement	Outcome measurement	Outcome valuation
Cost analysis	Pounds	Assumed identical	None
Cost-effectiveness analysis	Pounds	Single common specific variable	Common units (e.g. life years)
Cost-utility analysis	Pounds	All effects of the competing therapies	QALYs
Cost-benefit analysis	Pounds	All effects of the therapy evaluated	Pounds

Cost or cost-minimisation analysis (CMA)

This is the most simple form that an evaluation can take, as only the costs and not the benefits of a technology are compared. The implicit assumption of this form of analysis is that there is evidence that technologies are of equal effectiveness. As this is seldom likely with antihypertensive therapies it is questionable whether this form of analysis will be appropriate.

Cost-effectiveness analysis (CEA)

This involves comparing both the costs and outcomes of alternative technologies. Outcome is assessed in natural units. These can be related to what could be called patient outcomes (e.g. life years gained) or more clinical outcomes (e.g. reduction in mmHg). A technology is considered cost-effective if the cost per outcome achieved (e.g. cost per life year gained) is lower than the alternatives available.

Cost-utility analysis (CUA)

This is similar to CEA as alternatives are compared on the basis of cost per outcome achieved. However, in a CUA, outcome is measured in terms of the utility gained from treatment. Utility is generally equated to quantity of life weighted by quality of life. The most common measure of utility employed in studies is the quality adjusted life year or QALY (Gudex and Kind, 1988). In the evaluation of antihypertensive medications the consideration of quality, as well as quantity, of life can be seen as crucial. One of the major positive effects of therapy can be the reduction in non-fatal stroke and thus an improvement in quality rather than quantity of life. Similarly, a major disadvantage of therapy can be the detriment to quality of life caused by the side effects of treatment.

Cost-benefit analysis (CBA)

The above forms of analysis compare the costs of a technology to the benefits gained but do not address the question of whether or not the benefits of technologies outweigh their costs. In *cost-benefit analysis* all the costs and benefits of technologies are measured in monetary terms. Thus, alternatives can be compared by their absolute values – i.e. the monetary value of benefits less their cost. However, the application of CBA has been limited by methodological and ethical difficulties in measuring health gain in monetary terms.

Methodological requirements of economic evaluations

Table 8.2 details various principles to which economic evaluations should adhere (Coyle and Davies, 1993). These principles must be used for studies to have a relevance in any decisions to be made over the appropriateness of treatment.

It is important when assessing the quality of a study to be able to identify what question is addressed by the study. Economic evaluations of treatment for hypertension can answer a variety of questions (Table 8.3) and it is necessary for the question being addressed to be made explicit so that decision-makers can assess the relevance of the study. It is also important that the viewpoint from which the

Table 8.2 Principles of economic evaluation

1. The study question perspective and design must be clearly stated.
2. The study should involve a comparison of at least two alternatives. The 'do nothing', the least costly and the most used options should be considered.
3. All relevant costs and benefits of the alternatives should be identified and appropriately valued.
4. The study should be of a sufficient sample size to assess any significant differences between alternatives.
5. The marginal costs and benefits of alternatives should be valued.
6. Future costs and benefits should be appropriately discounted.
7. Detailed sensitivity analysis should be conducted.

Source: Coyle and Davies (1993)

Table 8.3 Questions that can be addressed by economic evaluation

1. What drug should we use in treating hypertension in the elderly?
   Which class of anti-hypertensive drug is most cost-effective?
2. Should we treat hypertension in the elderly with drug therapy?
   Is non-pharmacological treatment for hypertension cost-effective?
3. Should we take more steps to identify hypertensive patients?
   Is screening for hypertension in the elderly cost-effective?
4. Which hypertensive patients should we treat?
   For which characteristics of patients (e.g. sex, age, initial blood pressure) is treatment of hypertension more cost-effective?
5. Should we treat hypertension in the elderly?
   Is treatment of diastolic/systolic blood pressure greater than a certain level of mmHG cost-effective?

study is taken is made explicit. If this is unclear then decision-makers cannot be certain that the study will include all the costs and benefits of importance.

Evaluations must compare at least two alternative technologies; for example, two or more drug therapies for hypertension, or a non-pharmaceutical treatment programme and antihypertensive drug therapy. If only one technology is examined then no information will be gained about the relative cost-effectiveness of this technology. Also, it is vital that all relevant alternative treatments (i.e. all alternative drug therapies) are compared so that definitive conclusions over which is the most cost-effective technology available can be made.

In economic evaluations, the cost of a health technology should be measured by the resources necessary to introduce a technology into practice, i.e. the marginal cost. Economic evaluations, which include marginal costs, provide information to decision makers on the economic effect of providing health care interventions.

As, by nature, individuals prefer monetary benefits now rather than later and costs later rather than now, future costs and monetary benefits should be given reduced values to reflect this, i.e. they should be discounted. However, there is a lack of consensus over whether non-monetary (i.e. health) benefits should be similarly discounted (Coyle and Tolley, 1992). As the benefits of treatments for hypertension generally occur in the future – that is, extensions to the length of life, avoidance of non-fatal health problems – the issue of whether or not to discount future health benefits is of added importance. Coyle and Tolley (1992) have demonstrated that alternative discount rates for health benefits in the evaluation of antihypertensive agents lead to significant differences with regard to the conclusions of the analysis.

Finally, researchers conducting studies will not have perfect information on the costs and benefits of studies and will, therefore, have to make assumptions concerning certain factors. In evaluating treatments for hypertension, as benefits generally occur in the future, assumptions over the effects of therapy must be made. Where such assumptions have been made, it is essential that evaluations contain analyses which test the sensitivity of study results to changes in these assumptions.

Model for assessing the cost-effectiveness of treatment for hypertension

Stason and Weinstein (1977) created a model from which all forms of treatment for hypertension can be assessed in terms of their cost-effectiveness. They identified the following key components which needed to be considered:

- Costs of therapy (drugs plus monitoring)
- Costs of treating coronary heart disease (CHD)/stroke
- Costs of treating side effects of therapy
- Compliance with therapy
- Increase in survival due to a reduction in fatal CHD/stroke
- Improvements in quality of life due to a reduction in non-fatal CHD/stroke
- Effects of therapy on quality of life, i.e. side effects.

Allowing for these components, a formula was constructed from which the cost-effectiveness of treatments can be assessed:

$$\frac{C}{E} = \frac{\Delta C_{RX} - \Delta C_{MORB} + \Delta C_{SE}}{\Delta Y + \Delta Y_{MORB} - \Delta Y_{SE}}$$

Key

C = Total costs of treatment
ΔC_{RX} = Additional costs of (drug) treatment
ΔC_{MORB} = Reduction in costs of treating morbidity
ΔC_{SE} = Costs of treating side effects

E = Total benefits from treatment
ΔY = Years of life gained
ΔY_{MORB} = Improved quality of life due to reduced morbidity
ΔY_{SE} = Decrease in quality of life due to side effects of therapy

Source: Stason and Weinstein (1977).

This formula will generate costs per quality adjusted life years for each treatment option and thus the most cost-effective option can be identified. The incremental cost per QALY gained of treatment can also be compared to other interventions for other diseases to assess whether antihypertensive therapy is worthwhile.

COSTS AND BENEFITS RELATED TO THE TREATMENT OF HYPERTENSION

Costs of treatment

The cost of therapy, at first sight, appears to be the most dominant of all the components in assessing cost-effectiveness. The wide variation in the costs of drug therapy is illustrated in Table 8.4. Diuretics and beta-blockers are apparently the least costly of the drug classes recommended for long-term use in elderly patients.

Of interest is the difference in cost between generic and branded drugs. Although newer classes of drugs such as angiotensin-converting enzyme inhibitors (ACE inhibitors) and calcium channel blockers are currently more expensive, the ending of patent protection may lead to reduced costs for these drug classes due to increased price competition with generic manufacturers. Thus, merely concluding that the older classes of drugs are less expensive than the newer alternatives does not allow for the possible effects of a more dynamic market for the other drug classes after the end of patent protection.

The yearly costs of long-term drug mono-therapies ranges from a very cheap £1.65 to the high figure of £340 per annum. In the UK, additional life expectancy at age 65 is currently 14.3 years for males and 18.1 years for females (Department of Health, 1994a). Therefore, lifetime costs of drug therapy alone for hypertension in the elderly can be as much as £5000 for males and £6200 for females. In addition, one must allow for the annual costs of GP consultations with respect to hypertension. The current cost of a GP surgery consultation in the UK is £7.62 (Netten and Smart, 1993) and with patients possibly having consultations at least

Table 8.4 Annual costs of antihypertensive therapy (UK £1994)

	Cost per minimum dose*	Cost per maximum dose*
Diuretics		
Generic	1.65	1.65
Branded	3.65–7.76	15.51–16.79
Beta-blockers		
Generic	5.07–79.30	9.10–130.26
Branded	28.47–117.26	57.07–163.28
Alpha-adrenoceptor blocking agents		
Generic	44.33–137.28	183.04–259.48
Branded	44.33–137.28	183.04–259.48
ACE inhibitors		
Generic	143.39–156.39	266.50–340.60
Branded	143.39–156.39	266.50–340.60
Calcium channel blockers		
Generic	25.09–134.68	109.20–334.88
Branded	99.71–134.68	249.08–334.88

*Minimum and maximum doses as defined in the British National Formulary (British Medical Association, 1994)

every 2 months, the additional costs will be at least £45 – in many cases greater than the actual cost of the drugs prescribed. Given the magnitude of these figures and the incidence of hypertension in the elderly, it is perhaps not surprising that there is concern for containing the costs of antihypertensive therapy.

An alternative to drug therapy for elderly hypertensives is various forms of non-pharmacological treatments such as diet and exercise. In the most detailed study of the costs of non-pharmacological treatment for hypertension, conducted in Sweden (Johannesson *et al.*, 1991), a non-pharmacological treatment programme of regular consultations by health professionals, exercise, dietary advice, and home blood pressure measurements cost up to SEK 5300 (1 SEK = approximately £10) more than the average costs of drug therapies.

No specific study of the costs of non-drug treatment for hypertension in the UK has been conducted. However, assuming therapy would consist each month of visits by district nurses to measure blood pressure, GP consultations, National Health Service physiotherapy and dietary advice, the annual costs of such a programme would be as high as £500 (based on cost data from Netten and Smart, 1993). Therefore, it is likely that non-pharmacological treatment for hypertension will be initially of greater cost than pharmacological treatment.

Costs averted through treatment

Although the lifetime costs of therapy may appear high, these must be considered alongside the reductions in medical costs as a result of reduced fatal and non-fatal events. Treatment of hypertension in the elderly can lead to benefits in terms of reduced morbidity (non-fatal cerebrovascular disease (CVD) and non-fatal CHD) and reduced mortality (fatal CVD and CHD).

It is possible only to give rough estimates of the costs of treating fatal and non-fatal CVD and CHD in the UK. The average length of stay for a hospital admission for CVD and acute myocardial infarction in the UK in 1992–93 were 28.8 days and 9.8 days respectively (Department of Health, 1994b), with an estimated cost per bed day of £156 (based on Department of Health, 1994b). Thus, the hospital care for patients per CVD event and per acute myocardial infarction can be estimated to be £4493 and £1529 respectively.

For patients with non-fatal events there are likely to be additional medical costs (e.g. stroke rehabilitation, drug therapy) associated with morbidity. No accurate estimates of the costs of treating patients with non-fatal CVD or CHD in the UK exist. In the UK in 1985 there were estimated to be 320 000 patients contacting their GP with the primary diagnosis of cerebrovascular disease at a total cost to the National Health Service of £550 million (Dale, 1988). Adjusting for inflation, the current annual medical care costs per CVD patient are estimated to be £3190. No similar figure can be estimated for non-fatal CHD, although it is likely to be of approximately the same magnitude.

Benefits from treatment

The assessment of the benefit of treatment in terms of reducing coronary heart disease and stroke is problematic due to the long-term nature of therapy. Thus, most evaluations have based their estimates either on single clinical trials [e.g. the European Working Party on Hypertension in the Elderly (Amery *et al.*, 1985) or the Swedish Trial of Old Patients with Hypertension (Dahlof *et al.*, 1993), overviews of clinical trials (e.g. Collins *et al.*, 1990) and population surveys (e.g. the Framingham Heart Study – Kannel and Gordon, 1974]. The evidence on the benefits of treating hypertension in the elderly is covered elsewhere in this volume.

Similarly, allowance for the effects on quality of life, both in terms of reduced morbidity and side effects from therapy, is problematic within an economic evaluation. A large body of literature exists on the quality of life of hypertensives on therapy (Croog *et al.*, 1986; Fletcher *et al.*, 1990) and again is discussed elsewhere in this volume. However, few studies have attempted to measure the quality of life effects in terms of utility. Thus, CUAs of hypertensive therapy have tended to use *ad hoc* measures of the utility gained and lost through therapy.

A REVIEW OF THE COST-EFFECTIVENESS OF TREATMENT FOR HYPERTENSION IN THE ELDERLY

There have been a number of studies of the cost-effectiveness of treatment for hypertension in the general population, the most relevant of which are discussed below. The results of many of these studies have specific relevance when evaluating treatment of hypertension in the elderly population.

The study by Stason and Weinstein (1977) was the first study of the cost-effectiveness of treatment for hypertension. The study was a CUA examining the cost-effectiveness of drug treatment for patients of different age, sex and initial blood pressure. For men, the cost-effectiveness ratio increased with age whilst the opposite was the case with females. For both sexes, cost-effectiveness was greater the higher the level of pretreatment diastolic blood pressure.

The major problem with the study was the basis from which the benefits of therapy were measured. The study utilised data from the Framingham Study (Kannel and Gordon, 1974), as evidence from major clinical trials was limited at the time of analysis. Most studies since have used data from the various reported trials to model the benefits of therapy and have led to different results from the Stason and Weinstein study.

Burns (1989) considered the issues relating to the cost-effectiveness of treating hypertension specifically in the elderly. He identified a similar difference in the USA in the cost of treatment by the various drug classes and the cost savings to be made through generic pricing. Although not a formal analysis, after reviewing the available data on both the costs and effectiveness of treatment, Burns concluded that a carefully chosen stepped care regime can be inexpensive and cost-effective. The stepped care approach favoured by Burns involves initial daily treatment with 25 mg hydrochlorothiazide followed by reserpine or hydralazine (both 100 mg daily) in non-responders. The cost per death averted under this stepped care approach was estimated to be US$3535 compared to US$46000 for initial treatment by calcium antagonists and US$31000 for initial treatment by ACE inhibitors. Wright (1988) in a review of existing evidence on costs and effectiveness of alternative approaches to the management of hypertension, similarly argued that a stepped care approach with thiazide diuretics as initial therapy was likely to be a more cost-effective strategy than initial adoption of more costly drug classes.

Edelson and colleagues (1990) conducted a CEA examining the relative cost-effectiveness of alternative drug classes as initial monotherapies for treating mild to moderate hypertension in the US through the years 1990 to 2010. The estimated cost per year of life saved for this period was $10 900 for propranolol, $16 400 for hydrochlorothiazide, $31 600 for nifedipine, $61 900 for prazosin and $72 100 for captopril. Thus, the conclusion of the study was that beta-blockers were the most cost-effective class of drugs. However, the study did not examine the cost-effectiveness of antihypertensive therapy by age or sex. Nor did the study adequately allow for differences between therapies in terms of their effects on quality of life – possibly a major factor in favour of the more costly drug classes.

Kawachi and Malcolm (1990) conducted a CUA to answer an alternative question – is antihypertensive therapy for various age–sex–initial blood pressure groups cost-effective? The study was concerned with drug therapy in general and did not examine the differences between drug classes. In this study benefit was expressed in quality adjusted life years gained, i.e. the authors allowed for both the effect of therapy and the effect of non-fatal events on the quality of life of patients. The study found that the lower the pre-treatment blood pressure the less cost-effective treatment was. Additionally, in contrast to the Stason and Weinstein study, it was found that the older the patient the more cost-effective therapy was. The implication of the study was that in many cases, especially for younger individuals with only mild hypertension, drug therapy was not cost-effective and resources could be better employed elsewhere. However, in most cases, treatment of hypertension for the elderly did appear cost-effective.

A CUA by Drummond and Coyle (1992) involved modelling data from the study by Kawachi and Malcolm to examine which drug class was most cost-effective for treating hypertensives with various age–sex–initial blood pressure characteristics. The drug classes examined were diuretics, first generation beta-blockers, calcium antagonists and ACE inhibitors. The major conclusions of the study were similar to the Kawachi and Malcolm study: i.e. treatment of older patients was more cost-effective than younger patients, treatment of men was more cost-effective than women and it was more cost-effective to treat patients with higher pre-treatment blood pressure. In most instances for both males and females aged over 60 assuming that quality of life on therapy was lower when receiving diuretics, beta-blockers were the most cost-effective initial monotherapy. If no differences in quality of life were assumed, diuretics would be the most cost-effective option. However, for patients with mild hypertension, the more expensive drug classes (calcium antagonists and ACE inhibitors) appeared to be as cost-effective.

The authors also examined the cost-effectiveness of a stepped care approach to treatment whereby individuals commenced treatment with the lower cost diuretics or beta-blockers but were prescribed ACE inhibitors or calcium antagonists if the side effects of therapy were too severe. The study concluded that for all patient groups the stepped care approach was most cost-effective. The authors concluded by emphasising that their study was exploratory and that more research was required for the accurate measurement of the effect on patient's utility from the benefits and side effects of therapy.

Two studies have considered the cost-effectiveness of treatment for hypertension other than drug therapy (Ginsberg *et al.*, 1993; Johannesson *et al.*, 1991). In the study by Johannesson and colleagues (1991), the cost-effectiveness of a non-drug treatment programme was compared with standard drug therapy. The non-drug programme examined consisted of regular visits from health professionals, dietary advice and encouragement of physical activity.

The study is the only available CBA of treatment for hypertension. The benefit of treatment was expressed in monetary terms by asking patients their willingness to pay for the treatment. The cost of the non-pharmaceutical treatment programme was estimated to be 5300 Swedish Kroner per patient while the mean willingness of patients to pay for the programme was 3200 Swedish Kroner. Thus the programme led to a societal loss of 2100 Swedish Kroner. The authors conclude that the non-drug programme was no more cost-effective than drug therapy although a prospective study comparing the alternatives was required.

The study by Ginsberg and colleagues (1993), although purporting to be a CBA, was a CMA in which the costs of two alternative programmes, involving nutritional advice, exercise and stress management, for the non-pharmacological control of hypertension were compared. The study concluded that both regimes were cost-effective as they reduced the costs of therapy with adequate control of blood pressure. However, this study focused only on hypertensives aged between 35 and 65 years old. Therefore, it is questionable whether the benefits of therapy found in this study would be replicated in an elderly population.

A recent study (Johannesson *et al.*, 1993) was concerned solely with assessing the cost-effectiveness of antihypertensive therapy in the elderly population. The study was conducted utilising data from the Swedish Trial in Old Patients with Hypertension (STOP-Hypertension) (Dahlof *et al.*, 1993). The STOP study involved 1627 hypertensive patients aged between 70 and 84 years old with a supine blood pressure of greater than or equal to 180/105 mmHg. Patients were randomised to either placebo or treatment by diuretic or beta-blocker. Patients were followed up for a period of 25 months from which estimates of the costs of therapy and the effects in terms of increased life expectancy were obtained. The main results of the economic evaluation were that antihypertensive therapy for men aged between 70 and 84 cost 5000 Swedish Kroner per life year saved and for women the cost was 15000 Swedish Kroner. The conclusion reached by the authors was that treatment of elderly hypertensives by diuretic or beta-blockers was significantly cost-effective when compared with the cost per life year saved of other clinical interventions.

A further study by Johannesson (1994) analysed the results of 19 randomised controlled trials with respect to the cost per life year gained from antihypertensive therapy. The authors adopted a regression analysis technique to explore the effect of age and initial diastolic blood pressure on the relative cost-effectiveness of therapy. The analysis showed a statistically significant decrease in the cost per life year gained of treatment, per year of older age, of SEK 16 000. The conclusion from this study was that the older the patient is, the more cost-effective antihypertensive therapy will be.

DISCUSSION

The costs of treating hypertension in the elderly are high, with non-pharmaco-logical treatment appearing to be no less expensive than long-term drug therapy. Although these costs appear relatively low compared to the medical costs of morbidity and mortality occurring due to hypertension, none of the analyses identified above found any instances where the costs of therapy could be offset by future cost savings. Thus, treatment of hypertension in the elderly provides benefits in reducing future morbidity and mortality, which must be contrasted to the net costs of antihypertensive therapy. When assessing the cost-effectiveness of antihypertensive therapy in the elderly it is necessary to consider both the benefits of treatment in terms of health improvements and cost savings as well as the direct treatment costs. Economic evaluation thus provides a systematic approach for assessing whether the benefits of treating hypertension in the elderly are worth the cost.

There is no definitive study of the cost-effectiveness of treating hypertension in the elderly. The results of available analyses are sensitive to changes to the range of factors, the quality of life on therapy, and the long-term benefits from therapy. Most studies aim to answer one of the questions detailed in Table 8.2. Hence, overall conclusions over the economic worth of treatments must be made through an overview of all published studies. However, the lack of evidence on the long-term effects of therapy on mortality and morbidity of all alternative interventions means that the conclusions drawn from the studies must be seen as tentative. More research of a long-term nature is required and must focus on effects, quality of life and costs before definitive statements on cost-effectiveness of alternative treatments can be made. However, despite their limitations, the published studies tend to reach similar conclusions.

With respect to question 1 of Table 8.2, the lack of detailed information on the long-term benefits of different drug classes with respect to quality of life on therapy, as well as improvements in morbidity and mortality, make any conclu-sions over which drug class is most cost-effective very tenuous. No published study addressing this issue with regard to treatment of the elderly is available. However, most studies support the use of a stepped care approach in the manage-ment of hypertension in the elderly. Diuretics and beta-blockers, considerably the least expensive classes of drugs, are also the most cost-effective initial monotherapies for the treatment of hypertension and more expensive drug classes are only recommended if these drugs cannot be tolerated.

With respect to question 2, there is no evidence to indicate, given the evidence from available studies, that non-pharmacological treatment is more cost-effective than drug therapy in the treatment of elderly patients. There is also no evidence on which to base any conclusions regarding whether screening elderly patients for hypertension is cost-effective.

With respect to question 4, most studies conclude that treating hypertension in the elderly is considerably more cost-effective than treating younger patients. In general it has been found that cost-effectiveness improves the older the patient (Johannesson and Jonssön, 1991) and thus treatment of the elderly should be given high priority (Kawachi, 1994). This is primarily because the older the patient, the quicker the benefits of therapy in terms of life extension occur, and the lower the costs of long-term therapy due to the lower life expectancy of patients.

Finally, with respect to question 5, most studies conclude that in comparison with the costs and benefits of other clinical interventions, the pharmacological treatment of hypertension in the elderly is a cost-effective use of scarce resources.

REFERENCES

Amery A, Birkenhager W, Brixko P *et al*. 1985. Mortality and morbidity results from the European Working Party on high blood pressure in the elderly trial. *Lancet* **i**, 1349–54.

Backhouse ME, Backhouse RJ, Edey SA 1992. Economic evaluation bibliography. *Health Economics* **1**(Suppl.), 1–236.

British Medical Association 1994. *British National Formulary*. London: The Pharmaceutical Press.

Burns R 1989. Cost effectiveness in the treatment of hypertension. *Clinics in Geriatric Medicine* **5**, 829–40.

Collins R, Peto R, MacMahon S *et al*. 1990. Blood pressure, stroke and coronary heart disease. Part 2, short-term reductions in blood pressure: overview of randomised drug trials in their epidemiological context. *Lancet* **335**, 827–38.

Commonwealth of Australia 1992. *Guidelines for the pharmaceutical industry on preparation of submissions to the Pharmaceutical Benefits Advisory Committee, including submissions involving economic analyses*. Canberra: Department of Health, Housing and Community Services.

Coyle D, Davies L 1993. How to assess cost-effectiveness: elements of a sound economic evaluation. In Drummond M, Maynard AK (eds) *Purchasing and providing cost-effective health care*. London: Churchill Livingstone.

Coyle D, Tolley K 1992. Discounting of health benefits in the pharmacoeconomic analysis of drug therapies. An issue for debate? *Pharmacoeconomics* **2**, 153–62.

Croog SH, Levine S, Testa MA *et al*. 1986. The effects of antihypertensive therapy on quality of life. *New England Journal of Medicine* **314**, 1657–64.

Dahlof B, Hansson L, Lindholm LH, Schersten B, Ekbom T, Wester PO 1993. Swedish trial in old patients with hypertension (STOP-Hypertension) analyses performed up to 1992. *Clinical and Experimental Hypertension* **15**, 925–39.

Dale S 1988. *Stroke*. London: Office of Health Economics.

Department of Health 1994a. *Health and personal social services statistics for England*. London: HMSO.

Department of Health 1994b. *Hospital episodes systems*, Vol. 1, 1992–93. London: HMSO.

Drummond M, Coyle D 1992. Assessing the economic value of antihypertensive medicines. *Journal of Human Hypertension* **6**, 495–501.

Drummond MF, Stoddart GT, Torrance GW 1987. *Methods for economic evaluation of health care programmes*. Oxford: Oxford University Press.

Edelson JT, Weinstein MC, Tosteson ANA, Williams L, Lee TH, Goldman L 1990. Long-term cost-effectiveness of various initial monotherapies for mild to moderate hypertension. *Journal of the American Medical Association* **263**, 408–13.

Fletcher AE, Bulpitt CJ, Hawkins CM *et al*. 1990. Quality of life on antihypertensive therapy: a randomized double-blind controlled trial of captopril and atenolol. *Journal of Hypertension* **9**, 463–6.

Ginsberg GM, Viskoper JR, Fuchs Z *et al*. 1993. Partial cost-benefit analysis of two different modes of nonpharmacological control of hypertension in the community. *Journal of Hypertension* **7**, 593–7.

Gudex C, Kind P 1988. *The QALY toolkit*. Centre for Health Economics Discussion Paper 38. York: University of York.

Johannesson M 1994. The impact of age on the cost-effectiveness of hypertension treatment – an analysis of randomised drug trials. *Medical Decision Making* **14**, 236–44.

Johannesson M, Aberg H, Agreus L, Borgquist L, Jonsson B 1991. Cost-benefit analysis of non-pharmacological treatment of hypertension. *Journal of Internal Medicine* **230**, 307–12.

Johannesson M, Dahlof B, Lindholm LH *et al*. 1993. The cost-effectiveness of treating hypertension in elderly people – an analysis of the Swedish Trial in Old Patients with Hypertension (STOP Hypertension). *Journal of Internal Medicine* **234**, 317–23.

Johannesson M, Jonssön B 1991. Cost-effectiveness analysis of hypertension treatment: a review of methodological issues. *Health Policy* **19**, 55–77.

Kannel WB, Gordon T (eds) 1974. *The Framingham study: An epidemiological investigation of cardiovascular disease, section 30*. Washington DC: Government Printing Office.

Kawachi I 1994. Epidemiology of stroke. Importance of preventive pharmacological strategies in elderly patients and associated costs. *Drugs and Aging* **5**, 288–99.

Kawachi I, Malcolm LA 1990. Treating mild to moderate hypertension: cost-effectiveness and policy implications. *Journal of Cardiovascular Pharmacology* **16**(Suppl. 7), S126–8.

Netten A, Smart S 1993. *Unit Cost of Community Care 1992/93*. Canterbury: University of Kent Personal Social Services Research Unit.

Ontario Ministry of Health 1994. *Ontario guidelines for economic analyses of pharmaceutical products*. Toronto: Ministry of Health.

Robertson JI 1989. Hypertension and its treatment in the elderly. *Clinical and Experimental Hypertension – Part A, Theory and Practice* **11**, 779–805.

Shaw J 1993. High blood pressure–current state of play. *Australian Family Physician* **22**, 702–6.

Stason WB, Weinstein MC 1977. Allocation of resources to manage hypertension. *New England Journal of Medicine* **296**, 732–9.

Whitcomb B, Byyny RL 1990. Perspective on hypertension in the elderly. *Western Journal of Medicine* **152**, 392–400.

Wright JT Jr 1988. Geriatric hypertension therapy: a guide to cost-effectiveness. *Geriatrics* **43**, 55–62.

CHAPTER 9

The effects of antihypertensive therapy on psychomotor performance, quality of life, symptoms and laboratory parameters

DAN R LEE AND STEPHEN HD JACKSON ─────────────────────────

INTRODUCTION

Since 1964 when Michael Hamilton published his observations on the benefits of therapy (Hamilton *et al.*, 1964), treatment of hypertension has been aimed at reducing the risk of life-threatening complications. Since then, the threshold for treating hypertension has gradually fallen, the age above which treatment is not routinely offered has risen and the range of treatments available has dramatically enlarged. There remains uncertainty as to whether the benefit of reduction in vascular complications is a consequence of blood pressure reduction, regardless of method used. However, ongoing trials should resolve this. Differences in adverse reactions between drugs have become more relevant considerations than they were 10 years ago. Adverse events were traditionally documented as changes in laboratory variables, development of physical signs (e.g. rash) or response to questions about specific physical symptoms. In this way the rise in serum uric acid during thiazide diuretic treatment was demonstrated in excess of that during placebo therapy. Similarly, the excess prevalence of ankle swelling during nifedipine therapy and the excess prevalence of sexual dysfunction in men taking both thiazides and beta-blockers were identified in these ways.

The next stage in the evolution of the methodology for the characterisation of antihypertensive effects was the development of methods for objective measurement of mental functioning (psychomotor performance) and examining effects on patients' perception of their physical and mental well-being (quality of life). Quality of life (QOL) is perhaps best regarded as a concept rather than as a specific entity. Calman (1984), in another context, described quality of life as the gap between patients' expectations and achievements. The instruments that have been developed for use in patients with hypertension have focused on a number of main areas or domains: global well-being, physical symptoms (including sexual dysfunction), physical activity and psychological well-being/distress. Although of relevance to younger patients, work performance scales are not of wide relevance to patients above retirement age, although social interaction measures are useful. Objective measurements of mental function include tests of memory, central processing, integration and motor responses.

Mental functions should be regarded as a hierarchy, just as cortical sensory function (e.g. astereognosis – two-point discrimination) cannot be assessed in the presence of a lower sensory deficit, so attention and concentration cannot be assessed in the presence of sedation. Thus a drug such as methyldopa, which has significant sedative effects, will inevitably produce changes in a variety of psychomotor performance (PP) tests. Similarly, QOL assessments during treatment with antihypertensives known to cause, for example, gout, diabetes or wheeze should pick up the effects such agents will inevitably have on QOL.

As with any test, QOL instruments and PP tests should ideally be valid (should measure what they are supposed to measure), repeatable (give the same answer on repeat testing) and sensitive to change (in this case be able to detect drug effects). The demonstration of validity where there is no gold standard is always difficult and unsatisfactory. 'Validation' of tests under these circumstances is usually based on whether the test can reasonably be expected to measure the function it is supposed to measure and whether the results are similar to other tests of the same function. Thus, although QOL and PP tests have been developed that assure repeatability and sensitivity, validation is not quite as well demonstrated.

Confounding variables affecting the interpretation of the effects of antihypertensive therapy on brain function include the effects of both hypertension itself and the structural effects of cerebrovascular disease consequent upon hypertension.

The published literature on the effects on PP and QOL of the treatment of hypertension in elderly patients is limited. This chapter is not seeking to provide a meta-analysis, particularly as the methodological differences are great. References to published work, therefore, are not restricted to those that might qualify for inclusion in a meta-analysis. Much of the published work referred to in the text is summarised in table form: PP in Table 9.1 and QOL in Table 9.2.

PSYCHOMOTOR PERFORMANCE

Terminology

The terminology used in describing sensory input, the organisation and storage of information and motor response is confusing and is often applied loosely to describe concepts. Definitions of the commonly used terms are therefore important.

The term *psychomotor performance* refers to an assessment of the efficiency in the execution of mental processes and their consequent motor response. However, since testing these processes inevitably involves measuring a reaction to a specific stimulus, the phrase is used here to refer globally to the whole process of the reception of a sensory stimulus, its organisation, interpretation and storage and the motor response to it.

The terms *cognitive function* and *intellectual function* are variously used either globally in the same way as PP above or can be used to refer specifically to mental processes.

General considerations

Published data on the effects of hypertension and antihypertensive treatment on PP spanning the last 50 years have concentrated primarily on middle-aged patients. Results obtained from studies in younger hypertensives cannot readily be extrapolated to elderly hypertensives because scores on PP tests are age dependent as are the pharmacokinetics of the drugs used.

It is particularly important to define drug induced changes in PP in elderly patients because as a group they suffer a greater incidence of adverse drug reactions than do young patients, which is a particularly important factor in an asymptomatic condition such as uncomplicated hypertension. As a group, elderly patients have a more limited cognitive reserve than younger patients and therefore prescribers need to be especially aware of the PP effects of the drugs they use.

Some studies have concentrated on an older population but comparisons between studies are difficult because of widely differing methodologies. Many studies have been poorly controlled, particularly for co-existent cerebrovascular disease which can be responsible for impairment of PP independent of blood pressure. Various definitions of hypertension have been used and different degrees of blood pressure fall obtained. Some of the PP tests used have not been validated in terms of sensitivity to detection of small improvements in PP in elderly patients and most have not built a prestudy training period for PP tests into the study design to eliminate practise effects, which may in themselves account for improvement in scores over time.

Studies not controlling for drug class

A number of studies have looked at the general effect of treating hypertension on PP in elderly patients without being able to draw conclusions on individual treatments.

The Framingham study examined the relationship between blood pressure, antihypertensive treatment and PP in a descriptive manner in 2032 subjects examined between 1976 and 1978, and initially reported no relationship between blood pressure and PP, nor antihypertensive treatment and PP (Farmer *et al.*, 1987). However, blood pressure was only assessed on one occasion and took no account of chronicity of hypertension. When the data were re-analysed to include the proportion of visits classified as hypertensive over the previous 26 years, the authors found that in the untreated group a high blood pressure was associated with a poor PP although no association was found in the treated group (Farmer *et al.*, 1990). In addition, an association was found between poor PP and

Table 9.1 Studies examining the relationship between antihypertensive treatment and psychomotor performance (PP) in elderly patients

Age	Patients	Study design	PP tests	Treatments (mg)	Conclusions	Comments	Reference
55–89	n = 1993 (1356 off treatment) HT=BP>159/94	Longitudinal population study (not an interventional study)	LMIR, LMDR, VR, PAL, DF, DB, WF, S	Not stated	• No relationship between either BP or antihypertensive treatment and PP	• Framingham cohort • HT based purely on one assessment and therefore likely to have included white-coat hypertensives • No comment on specific treatments	Farmer et al., 1987
55–89	As above	As above + Proportion of assessments classified as hypertensive compared to PP in treated and untreated groups	As above	Not stated	• High proportion of hypertensive assessments associated with poorer PP in untreated group • No association between BP and PP in treated group	• Reanalyis of Framingham cohort • Observational nature makes interpretation impossible	Farmer et al., 1990
>60	n = 551 (108 placebo) SBP 160–219 DPB< 90	Randomised, placebo-controlled, parallel group	SHORT-CARE, DSST, TMT, DSS	Chlorthalidone (12.5–25) ± atenolo/reserpine Placebo	• Weak negative association between SBP and PP at baseline • No association after 1 year of treatment	• Subgroup of SHEP • Treatment effect on PP potentially masked by coprescribing of reserpine, metoprolol or hydralazine • No significant fall in DBP observed	Gurland et al., 1988
65–74	n = 2401 SBP>160 DBP <113	Single-blind, randomised, placebo-controlled, parallel group study. Community based	NART, RM, PALT, TMT, DQ	Atenolol (50) Coamilozide (25/2.5) Placebo	• No adverse effect of treatment over 9 months • No differential effect on blood pressure between treatments	• MRC Treatment Trial of mild Hypertension in Older Adults • Difficulty in standardising PP test administration by 220 nurses	Bird et al., 1990

Age	Sample	Study design	Cognitive tests	Drugs	Findings	Comments	Reference
>60	n = 690, Males, SBP<240, DBP 90–114	Double-blind, randomised, placebo washout, parallel group	TMT, SDMT, TE, WMS, BVRT, VF		• Improvement in PP in both diuretic group and n = 55 placebo 'practice effect' control group • No difference in blood pressure or PP effect between low and high dose diuretic	• Improvement in both groups likely to be practise effect	Goldstein et al., 1990
60–81	n = 25, DBP 90–110	Double-blind, randomised, cross-over	BSRT, SWT, BD, DSST, VT, TMT, FT, RM	Atenolol (50–100), Nifedipine (30–90)	• Memory and complex abilities impaired in nifedipine group • No significant change in PP in atenolol group	• Results based on first arm of study only (scores did not return to baseline during second placebo phase)	Skinner et al., 1992
60–78	n = 23, Males, DBP 95–105	Double-blind, randomised, placebo-controlled, cross-over study	ART, BVRT, TMT, VF	Propranolol (20–80 bd)	• PP impairment associated with propranolol	• Pre-existing cerebrovascular disease not excluded • BP falls not reported	Kostis et al., 1990
75–85	n = 487, HT = SBP>160 or DBP >90	Observational study	BMT, ZDS, OA, DSST, DgS, PPT	Beta-blockers, Diuretics, Methyldopa	• No significant difference between treated HT and NT	• Bronx Aging Study • Unblinded and no placebo control • Cerebrovascular disease not excluded • No PP test training	Wurzelmann et al., 1987
>55	n = 17, HT = a documented high BP within past year	Double-blind, placebo-controlled, cross-over study	FT, SRT, DRT, CPT, TMT, SRemT (automated tests)	Hydrochlorothiazide (25), Propranolol LA (120), Enalapril (10)	• Diuretics associated with improved discriminate reaction time	• Most 'hypertensives' had DBP<90 mmHg at end of placebo phase • No significant BP fall obtained	McCorvey et al., 1993
61–79	n = 25, HT = SBP>165 & DBP>95	Single-blind, randomised, placebo-controlled, parallel group study. Cerebrovascular disease and dementia excluded	SDST, CAT, PWAT, CRT, CFF, INSP	Hydrochlorothiazide/triamterene (25+50), Captopril (25 bd), Nifedipine (20 bd), Atenolol (50 bd)	• Treatment associated with improvement in 4/6 tests • Improvement seen within 1 week of commencing treatment • Treatment groups too small to comment on specific drug effects	• PP tests automated and observer independent • PP training undertaken to eliminate practise effects	Kalra et al., 1993a

Table 9.1 *contd*

Age	Patients	Study design	PP tests	Treatments (mg)	Conclusions	Comments	Reference

61–79	n = 13
	HT = SBP>165 &
	DBP>95
		Double-blind,
		randomised,
		cross-over study.
		Cerebrovascular
		disease and dementia
		excluded
			SDST, CAT,
			PWAT, CRT,
			CFF
				Captopril (25 bd)
				Nifedipine (20 bd)
					• Both treatments
					  improved PP in
					  4/5 tests
					• No difference
					  between treatments
						• Improvement seen
						  within 1 week of
						  commencing
						  treatment
							Kalra et al., 1993a

>50	n = 50 HT
	n = 30 NT
	also studied young
	group (n = 50 HT
	= 50 NT)
	HT = DBP≥95–114
		Retrospective	VRT, PSS, CFF,
			TFFT, DSST,
			BD, TE, DM,
			JTL/JRT, FT,
			TCS, TT, MRT
				Diuretics
				Beta-blockers
				Centrally acting drugs
				(alone or in combination)
					• PP worse in HT
					  compared to NT
					• PP worse in elderly
					  compared to young
						• Individual treatment
						  effects not studied
						  in elderly
						• Retrospective design
						  limits interpretation
							Shapiro et al., 1989

55–90
mean = 63
	n = 27
	DBP≥95
		Double-blind, 3-way
		placebo-controlled,
		cross-over
			CFF, TMT,
			VAS – lethargy
				Metoprolol (150)
				Atenolol (100)
					• PP improvement
					  with both drugs
					• No effect of
					  lipophilicity on PP
					• Improved PP
					  coincides with
					  Cmax of both drugs
						• Built-in pre-study PP
						  test training
						  minimises
						  improvement during
						  active phase due to
						  practise effects
						• Only study to
						  correlate PP with
						  plasma concentration
						  of drug
							Gengo et al., 1988

≥65
mean = 70
	n = 242 females
	DBP≥95 & ≤114
	DBP = 95–114
		Double-blind,
		randomised, placebo
		run-in parallel group
			DSST, RAVLT,
			CFT, TCFT,
			TSW
				Diltiazem S/R (60–180 bd)
				Atenolol (50–100)
				Enalapril (5–20)
					• No adverse effect of
					  treatment on PP
					  (tendency towards
					  improvement)
						• Females only studied
						• No PP test training
							Applegate et al.,
							1991

Key to psychomotor performance tests and scales: ART – Auditory Retention Test; **BD** – Block Design; **BMT** – Blessed Mental Test; **BSRT** – Benton Selective Reminding Test; **BVRT** – Benton Visual Retention Test; **CAT** – Continuous Attention Test; **CFF** – Critical Flicker Frequency; **CFT** – Complex Figure Test; **CPT** – Continuous Performance Test; **CRT** – Choice Reaction Time; **DB** – Digits Backwards; **DgS** – Digit Span; **DF** – Digits Forwards; **DM** – Design Memory; **DQ** – Depression Questionnaire; **DRT** – Discriminant Reaction Time; **DS** – Dementia Scale; **DSS** – Double Simultaneous Stimulation; **DSST** – Digit Symbol Substitution Test; **FT** – Finger Tapping; **INSP** – Inspection Time; **LJRT** – Lift & Jump Reaction Time; **LMDR** – Logical Memory Delayed Recall; **LMIR** – Logical Memory Immediate Recall; **MRT** – Movement Reversal Time; **NART** – Nelson Adult Reading Test*; **OA** – Object Assembly; **PALT** – Paired Associate Learning Test; **PPT** – Purdue Pegboard Test; **PSS** – Perception of Spaced Stimuli; **PWAT** – Paired Word Association Test; **RAVLT** – Rey Auditory Verbal Learning Test; **RM** – Ravens Matrices; **S** – Similarities; **SDMT** – Symbol Digit Modalities Test; **SDST** – Symbol Digit Substitution Test; **SRemT** – Selective Reminding Test; **SRT** – Stimulus Reaction Time; **SWT** – Stroop Word Test; **TCS** – Transfer Coordination Speed; **TE** – Time Estimation; **TFFT** – Two Flash Fusion Test; **TMT** – Trail Making Test; **TSW** – Timed Sentence Writing; **TT** – Traverse Time; **VAS** – Visual Analogue Scale; **VF** – Verbal Fluency; **VR** – Visual Reproduction; **VRT** – Visual Recognition Threshold; **VT** – Vocabulary Test; **WF** – Word Flency; **WMS** – Wechsler Memory Scale being off treatment over the previous 2 years. This suggests that the time scale of the underlying mechanism is more rapid than the development of cerebrovascular disease.

Shapiro *et al.* (1989) examined, retrospectively, a group of patients aged >50 years who were attending a hypertension clinic (all of whom were on antihypertensive treatment) and compared their PP scores to age-matched normotensive controls. They found that the hypertensive group performed significantly worse than the normotensives and that their blood pressure was significantly greater than controls. They also studied a young hypertensive group with age-matched controls and concluded that PP in the young hypertensive group was similar to that in the old normotensive group. However, results of this study should be interpreted with caution in view of its retrospective design.

The Iowa 65+ Rural Health Study (Wallace *et al.*, 1985) investigated many facets of health and social functioning in a rural population. Reduced free recall memory in patients with diastolic hypertension was found whereas no such relationship was elicited with isolated systolic hypertension. The study was controlled for age, sex, educational attainment, antihypertensive drugs, alcohol, depression and physical activity, but not for hypertensive end-organ damage although patients with a history of stroke were excluded. Other psychomotor parameters were not measured, limiting further interpretation of this study.

Kalra *et al.* (1993a) studied PP in 25 hypertensives aged 61–79 years comparing scores after a placebo run-in period with those obtained after 1 and 4 weeks of antihypertensive therapy. They found that associated with a substantial fall in blood pressure (34/23 mmHg), PP improved within 1 week of commencing treatment and had not improved further by 4 weeks. This study excluded subjects with evidence of hypertensive end-organ damage and included a PP test prestudy training period. Although patients were randomised to one of five treatment groups (placebo + four active treatments), the numbers were too small to draw any conclusions on individual treatment effects.

The studies described above comment on the effect of antihypertensive treatment in general and do not draw any specific conclusions regarding the effects of individual treatments. These studies suggest that lowering blood pressure is associated with PP benefit in elderly patients with hypertension. However, a number of studies have investigated the effect of specific antihypertensive treatments on PP in elderly patients.

Diuretics

Diuretics are commonly prescribed for hypertension in elderly patients and although many studies have examined their effect on PP, few are specific to elderly patients.

A large study which arose from the Medical Research Council study of mild hypertension in elderly patients performed community-based testing on 2401 subjects and found no association between level of blood pressure at the outset of the study and cognitive function scores (Bird *et al.*, 1990). Two treatments were compared: a diuretic combination preparation (hydrochlorothiazide and amiloride) and a beta-blocker (atenolol). They commented that there was no difference between treatments in effect on PP with neither treatment adversely

Table 9.2 Studies reporting effects on QOL in older patients with hypertension (mean age >60 years)

Age	Patients	Study design	QOL measures	Treatments (mg)	Conclusions	Comments	Reference
60–79 mean = 68.8	n = 884 Blood pressure ≥170/105	Controlled comparison of active treatment versus nothing. Parallel group	Eight-symptom questionnaire	Atenolol (100) ± Bendrofluazide (5) ± Methyldopa	• No differences in symptoms were seen despite significant falls in blood pressure and cardiovascular endpoints	• Control group not given placebo • Eight-symptom questionnaire did not cover QOL	Coope and Warrender, 1986
≥60 mean = 72 in study as a whole	n = 551 (108 placebo) SBP 160–219 DPB< 90	Double-randomised, placebo-controlled, parallel group	SHORT-CARE		• No difference in SHORT-CARE scores between groups	• Subgroup of SHEP • SHORT-CARE covers depression, cognitive impairment, disability not QOL specifically	Gurland et al., 1988
≥60 mean = 72	n = 4736 SBP 160–219 DBP <90	Double-blind, randomised, placebo-controlled, parallel group	Questionnaires including SHORT-CARE, CES-D, ADLS, Social network	Chlorthalidone (12.5–25) ± Atenolol/reserpine Placebo	• No excess of any symptoms in placebo group • Active treatment associated with impaired memory/ concentration and sexual function	• Although symptom checklist covered the psychosocial domain, QOL not specifically reported	SHEP Co-operative Research Group, 1991
≥60 mean = 72	↑ ———— Follow up report on SHEP ———— ↓				• Both groups showed modest trend towards deterioration with time for more strenuous activities • Global QOL: no treatment effect • Depression scores: just reached significance in favour of active treatment	• No QOL disadvantage to treatment for isolated systolic hypertension	Applegate et al., 1994
≥60	n = 690 Males SBP<240 DBP 90–114	Double-blind, randomised, placebo-washout, parallel group	ADLS (modified CARE), ZDS	Low dose hydrochlorothiazide (25–50) High dose hydrochloro-thiazide (50–100) ± Hydralazine, methyldopa, metoprolol or reserpine	• No significant differences between low or high dose hydrochlorothiazide or between additional drug groups	• All patients received a thiazide making genuine comparison between groups difficult • Surprisingly, hydrochlorothiazide at any dose did not increase the frequency of problems with sexual activities	Goldstein et al., 1990

Age/mean	n and BP	Study design	QOL instruments	Drugs (doses)	Results	Comments	Reference
65–74 mean = 70	n = 2401 SBP 160–209 DBP ≤113 mean = 184/90	Double-blind, randomised, placebo-controlled, parallel group	SELF-CARE-D	Atenolol (50) Coamilozide (25/2.5) Placebo	• No differences in depression scores between the treatments	• MRC Treatment Trial of Mild Hypertension in Older Adults	Bird et al., 1990
>65 mean = 69	n = 28 SBP 160–209 DBP 95–115 mean = 181/102	Double-blind, randomised, placebo-washout, cross-over	Details not given	Bisoprolol (5–10) Captopril (50–100)	• No QOL differences	• Small sample size	Bracchetti et al., 1990
mean = 70	n = 242 women	Double-blind, controlled cross-over, randomised, dose-titration, parallel group	Psychological General Well-being Schedule and others	Atenolol (50–100) Enalapril (5–20) Diltiazem SR (120–360)	• No significant changes in QOL scores	• All treatments achieved a fall in blood pressure	Applegate et al., 1991
60–81 mean = 68	n = 31 BP mean = 166/97	Placebo washout, randomised, double-blind, cross-over	BDI, STAI, symptom inventory	Atenolol (25–100) Nifedipine (30–90)	• No effects of either drug on mood or anxiety • Ankle oedema and flushing more prevalent with nifedine	• Small sample size	Skinner et al., 1992
≥55 mean = 66	n = 17	Double-blind, randomised, placebo	Nottingham Health Profile	Hydrochlorothiazide (25) Propranolol ER (120) Enalapril (10) Placebo	• Propranolol and enalapril not significantly different using aggregated score on pt.1 NHP	• Sample size not large enough to show significant effect of active treatment on blood pressure • DBP in normotensive range on placebo in hypertensive group	McCorvey et al., 1993
55–79 mean = 64	n = 379 Males BP mean = 155/97	Placebo-washout, active treatment for 24 weeks	PD, PW, GPH, WWDR, SSD, SESDI, LEI, SI	Captopril 25–50 Enalapril 5–20 ± Hydrochlorothiazide	• BP and ADRs similar • Overall QOL (summary scale): captopril better than enalapril	• Higher baseline QOL patients worsened with enalapril but remained stable with captopril	Testa et al., 1993
60–80 mean = 68	n = 309 Females DBP 95–114 on placebo mean = 161/100	Placebo washout, randomised, double-blind	GWBAS, CES-D, STAI	Atenolol Enalapril Isradipine ± Hydrochlorothiazide	• No differences except cough was associated with enalapril and dry mouth with atenolol	Although the study was confined to women, the study methodology was appropriate. Good evidence of lack of effect	Croog et al., 1994

Key to QOL instruments: SHORT-CARE – Short Comprehensive Assessment and Referral Evaluation; SHORT-CARE-D – SHORT-CARE-Depression; CES-D – Center for Epidemiologic Studies – Depression Scale; ADLS – Activities of Daily Living Scale; ZDS – Zung Depression Scale; BDI – Beck Depression Inventory; STAI – State-Trait Anxiety Inventory; SELF-CARE-D – Self-rating Depression Questionnaire; GWBAS – General Well-Being Adjustment Scale; PSDI – Physical Symptoms Distress Index; SDI – Sleep Disturbance Index; VGH – Vitality General Health; SPAS – Social Participation Activities Scale; PD – Psychological Distress; PW – Psychological Well-being; GPH – General Perceived Health; WWDR – Well-being at Work or in Daily Routine; SSD – Sexual Symptom Distress; SESDI – Side Effects and Symptom Distress Index; LEI – Life Events Index; SI – Stress Index affecting PP within the first 9 months of antihypertensive treatment. However, a number of confounding issues make interpretation difficult. Once again the sensitivity of the test battery to minor CNS changes in elderly subjects was not presented, and the study group was not controlled for hypertensive end-organ damage. Inevitably in a community-based study, test conditions could not be standardised. There was also a suggestion that selection bias of subjects occurred as the mean IQ of the study group was 10 points higher than the national average, although this would not be expected to bias the effect of treatment on PP.

The Veterans study (Goldstein *et al.*, 1990) looked at PP in a group of elderly hypertensive males (690 men >60 years) in a double-blind, randomised, placebo-controlled design. Patients were treated with hydrochlorothiazide 25–100 mg daily as necessary with non-responders receiving in addition either hydralazine, methyldopa, metoprolol or reserpine. They also looked at a control group of elderly men matched for blood pressure who were not on treatment. They found that PP improved in the diuretic group but this improvement was no different to that of a control group. This change in PP in diuretic and control groups was ascribed to a practise effect making interpretation difficult. However, the authors concluded that since improvement was seen in both groups, the practise effect did not obscure a true deterioration on treatment. They also found that there was no difference in effect on PP between low and high dose diuretic and no significant difference in blood pressure fall (18/10 and 20/10 mmHg respectively). Interpretation of these results is further hampered by a failure to control adequately for coexistent cerebrovascular disease, which in itself may be responsible for impaired PP.

The SHEP (Systolic Hypertension in the Elderly Project) group measured PP in 443 treated isolated systolic hypertensives and 108 controls on placebo (Gurland *et al.*, 1988). This double-blind, randomised, placebo-controlled study measured PP and mood at baseline and after 1 year of treatment with chlorthalidone. They found a weak negative association between baseline systolic blood pressure and a composite PP score but no significant change in PP over 1 year despite a mean systolic blood pressure fall of 17 mmHg. Subjects with overt cerebrovascular disease and a recent myocardial infarction were excluded but training in PP tests was not undertaken. 12% of patients did not respond to diuretic alone, and received in addition either reserpine, metoprolol or hydralazine, which may have had a deleterious effect on any PP improvement.

McCorvey *et al.* (1993) compared the effect on blood pressure and PP of a diuretic (hydrochlorothiazide), beta-blocker (propranolol) and angiotensin-converting enzyme inhibitor (ACE inhibitor) (enalapril) on hypertensive patients over 55 years of age in a double-blind, placebo-controlled study. They found that the diuretic was associated with an improvement in tests of reaction time but not in other tests of cognitive function and PP. The other treatments were not associated with any significant change in any of the tests. However, patients were chosen on the basis of a history of hypertension and at the end of placebo run-in only one patient had a diastolic blood pressure >90 mmHg and in the active phase there was no significant diastolic blood pressure fall on any of the three treatments. The study was very small and in any event cannot be extrapolated to true hypertensives.

These studies suggest that treating elderly hypertensives with diuretics at least has no detrimental effect on PP and there is some evidence of a small beneficial effect.

Beta-blockers

This group of drugs has been the most extensively investigated in terms of effect on PP although again relatively few studies have focused on elderly patients.

Skinner *et al.* (1992) studied 25 elderly hypertensives in a double-blind, randomised cross-over study comparing the effect of atenolol versus nifedipine on a wide range of PP tests. Patients with cerebrovascular and cardiovascular disease as well as those with a history of depression or dementia were not included. Atenolol was associated with a significantly better score in the Buschke selective reminding test (a test of short-term memory) and DSST (a test of visuomotor co-ordination) when compared to nifedipine although not significantly different from placebo. However, in these tests, the scores did not return to baseline after the second placebo phase, suggesting either a carry-over effect from the first active treatment or inadequate PP test training and a consequent practise effect.

Applegate *et al.* (1991), in their study of effects on quality of life of atenolol, diltiazem and enalapril, also included a number of PP tests in their test battery. There were no adverse effects of treatment on PP and there was a tendency towards PP improvement on treatment. There was minimal difference between treatments in terms of PP effect although subjects on atenolol performed significantly worse on DSST at 8 weeks than did those on the other treatments. The significance of this difference, however, was lost by 16 weeks. This study was only carried out in women and cannot be extrapolated to elderly men.

The PP component of the Medical Research Council (MRC) study of hypertension in elderly patients (Bird *et al.*, 1990) has already been described under the diuretics section. Atenolol was also studied and was found to have no detrimental or beneficial effect on PP over the first 9 months of treatment and in this respect did not differ from hydrochlorothiazide and amiloride.

Kostis *et al.* (1990) studied 23 mild hypertensives aged 60–78 in a double-blind randomised placebo-controlled cross-over study looking at the effect of propranolol on a wide range of PP tests and found that propranolol was associated with a significant impairment of PP. Results were presented as a composite score based on weighted individual scores and the effect on specific cognitive functions was not described. The subjects were only very mildly hypertensive and no details of blood pressure fall achieved were given. No attempt was made to screen out subjects with hypertensive end-organ damage or a history of cerebrovascular disease. The relevance of the findings is therefore not at all clear.

The Veterans Administration study described above (Goldstein *et al.*, 1990) examined the effect of adding metoprolol to a diuretic regimen if blood pressure control was insufficient and concluded that this had no effect on PP although metoprolol was not studied independently.

Wurzelmann *et al.* (1987) studied PP in 487 hypertensives between the ages of 75 and 85 in an observational study. Patients were taking a range of antihypertensive medications but the group taking propranolol ($n = 48$) was large enough to warrant separate analysis. They found that propranolol had no effect on PP whereas a group taking benzodiazepines did significantly worse than controls. However, the study was not placebo-controlled and no test training was undertaken. The tests used were the Blessed Mental Test, a questionnaire developed for use in demented patients, and a small WAIS subset and the test battery's sensitivity to small changes in PP in hypertension had not been validated. Further, patients with cerebrovascular disease were not excluded, rendering this study useless.

Gengo *et al.* (1988) compared the effect on PP of metoprolol (a lipophilic beta-blocker) with atenolol (a hydrophilic beta-blocker) in a placebo-controlled, three-way cross-over study. They found that overall both drugs improved PP and there was no consistent effect of lipophilicity. On the study days, PP tests and serum samples for drug concentration were taken at hourly intervals and peak effect of PP improvement was found to coincide with the study drug maximum concentration.

In summary, studies variously suggest either an improvement or no significant effect of beta-blockers on PP in elderly hypertensives. One study described a detrimental effect of propranolol (Kostis *et al.*, 1990) but interpretation of this study is limited particularly because the patients were very mild hypertensives and the degree of blood pressure fall on treatment was not stated.

Calcium channel blockers

Only three studies have investigated the effects of calcium channel blocking agents in elderly patients with hypertension.

Skinner *et al.* (1992) studied the effect of both atenolol and nifedipine on PP in elderly hypertensives (as described under beta-blockers). Nifedipine was associated with a worsening of the Buschke Selective Reminding Test (a test of memory) and the Digit Symbol Substitution Test (a test of visuomotor co-ordination) and scored significantly worse than the scores attained by the atenolol group. However, the shortcomings of this study have already been described.

Kalra *et al.* (1993a) compared the effect on PP of nifedipine and an ACE inhibitor (captopril) in 13 elderly hypertensives in a double-blind cross-over study. The PP tests were a battery of automated tests which are sensitive to minor changes in PP. They found that nifedipine significantly improved a range of tests of memory, attention and central processing compared with baseline. Patients with evidence of hypertensive end-organ damage or dementia were excluded and all were trained to perform the tests until their performance reached a plateau prior to the active phase of the study in order to eliminate practise effects.

The details of a study comparing PP effects of atenolol, diltiazem and enalapril have already been described in the beta-blocker section (Applegate *et al.*, 1991). The analysis did not include significance testing for change from baseline for each individual treatment but diltiazem was associated with improvements in tests of central processing and memory. However, details of PP test training were not given, and these improvements could be explained by practise effects.

To date, there are no other studies that assess the effect on PP of calcium channel blockers in elderly patients although their use is increasing, particularly with the introduction of once-daily preparations. At present, the lack of data in this area makes conclusions regarding calcium channel blockers difficult to reach although there is evidence in favour of a beneficial effect on PP.

ACE inhibitors

Although some studies have looked at ACE inhibitors and PP in younger adults, only two have specifically studied their effects in elderly patients. Kalra *et al.* (1993a), as described above, compared PP effects of captopril with nifedipine in a double-blind cross-over study. They found captopril significantly improved tests of memory, attention and central processing but was not significantly different from nifedipine.

The study by Applegate *et al.* (1991) comparing diltiazem, atenolol and enalapril has already been described under the appropriate sections and found minimal difference in PP between groups. However, similarly to diltiazem, enalapril was associated with improvement in tests of central processing and memory although this may have been due in part to a practise effect.

Again, the paucity of data in this area makes conclusions difficult but both of these studies suggest that treating elderly hypertensives with ACE inhibitors is associated with improvement in PP.

Other antihypertensive medications

Antihypertensive drugs such as methyldopa, hydralazine, clonidine and reserpine were used extensively in the past but central effects with these drugs were common and they would be expected to cause impairment of PP independent of blood pressure. As newer drugs with a more acceptable side-effect profile have become available, their use has decreased.

The Bronx Aging study (Wurzelmann *et al.*, 1987), as described under betablockers, also studied methyldopa and found that it was associated with a significantly worse score on object assembly compared with the control group although other tests were unchanged. The shortcomings of this study have already been discussed. Studies involving younger patients confirm that methyldopa is associated with impairment of PP and a high incidence of adverse effects (Croog *et al.*, 1986; Solomen *et al.*, 1983).

Alpha-adrenergic blockers such as prazosin and doxazosin have fewer central effects than the drugs mentioned above but again can cause sedation. There is no published data on their effect on PP in any age group.

Conclusions

The studies concerning the relationship between blood pressure and PP in the elderly have used widely differing methodologies and have reached different conclusions. Although not reviewed here, most studies have shown impaired PP in hypertensives compared to normotensives (Kalra *et al.*, 1993b, 1994) and have either shown no effect or a small beneficial effect on PP of treating hypertension. Using drugs such as methlydopa, which are known to have a significant central action, in the treatment of hypertension in elderly patients leads to psychomotor impairment. Therefore it seems likely that lowering blood pressure in elderly hypertensives independently improves PP but this improvement can be offset by a direct, detrimental, central nervous system effect of the drugs used.

The explanation for the PP improvement on treating hypertension is not clear but the reversibility of the deficit within 1 week of commencing treatment demonstrated by Kalra *et al.* (1993) suggests the changes within the central nervous system are not structural but functional and reflect either a change in regional cerebral blood flow or an as yet undefined functional change at the cellular level. The clinical significance of these changes has not been demonstrated but it would be likely that, particularly in elderly patients who may have impaired psychomotor reserve, any impairment could lead to functional deterioration.

QUALITY OF LIFE

Introduction

Many scales have been used, of which most were developed for purposes other than the assessment of QOL in older hypertensive patients. The general health status measures that were at one time most widely used such as the Sickness Impact Profile (SIP) (Bergner *et al.*, 1981) and the Nottingham Health Profile (NHP) (Hunt, 1984) are probably not the most sensitive tools for use in a relatively asymptomatic patient group such as those with hypertension although they become more useful when complications develop. Of these, NHP is usually preferred because it is much quicker to administer than the SIP. As is apparent from Table 9.2, no QOL scale is widely used in the study of hypertension in older patients. The questionnaire proposed by Bulpitt and Fletcher (1990a) was developed in younger patients and has components investigating symptoms, psychological well-being and activity. It does not cover positive measures such as vitality or social participation. It has the advantage, however, of being suitable for self-administration, taking only 20–40 minutes to complete. Bowling (1995) has reviewed the available instruments.

Diuretics

Over a number of years three papers reporting the effects on QOL amongst patients recruited into the Systolic Hypertension in the Elderly Program (SHEP) have been published (Applegate *et al.*, 1994; Gurland *et al.*, 1988; SHEP Cooperative Research Group, 1991). The SHEP study was a randomised, placebo-controlled study of the treatment of isolated systolic hypertension that used chlorthalidone as the first-line agent with atenolol as the next choice treatment. The starting dose of 12.5 mg of chlorthalidone was increased to 25 mg if blood pressure was not controlled. The lack of effect of active treatment predominantly reflected the actions of chlorthalidone as approximately 50% of those randomised to active treatment received this drug alone. The main study randomised an impressive 4736 patients, contributing tremendous statistical power to the comparison between active treatment and placebo.

A number of symptoms were significantly more prevalent in the active treatment patients, e.g. trouble with memory/concentration and trouble with sexual function. Measures of cognitive and emotional function, however, did not differ between the groups (Applegate *et al.*, 1994). These measures were sensitive to change, demonstrating a modest deterioration with time in both groups.

The European Working Party on High Blood Pressure in the Elderly (EWPHE) study also employed a diuretic (hydrochlorothiazide and triamterene) as first-line active treatment in comparison with placebo (Amery *et al.*, 1985). As with other early interventional studies QOL was not formally measured, but the symptoms of dry mouth and diarrhoea both occurred more commonly in the active treatment group (Bulpitt and Fletcher, 1990b; Fletcher *et al.*, 1991). This excess seemed to be due to methyldopa, which was taken in addition to first-line therapy by one third of patients. Gout also occurred more frequently in the active treatment group with an incidence of four cases/1000 patients per year.

Goldstein *et al.* (1990), in a smaller study of 690 men with diastolic hypertension, compared low (25–50 mg) and high (50–100 mg) dose hydrochlorothiazide and found no differences on a range of subjective and objective tests (Table 9.2). Although this study employed a placebo washout phase prior to active treatment, there was no placebo control. The Hypertension Detection and Follow-up Program study performed in the United States compared stepped care treatment using chlorthalidone as the first-line drug, with referred care (Hypertension Detection and Follow-up Program Co-operative Group, 1979). No conclusions concerning the adverse effects of specific drug classes can be drawn but it is of interest that for all adverse reactions the incidence was lower in patients aged 60–69 compared with younger patients (Curb *et al.*, 1988).

The MRC trial of mild hypertension in older adults demonstrated no effect of hydrochlorothiazide on Depression Questionnaire scores (Bird *et al.*, 1990). It did, however, demonstrate a significant excess of withdrawals from hyperglycaemia, skin reactions, nausea and dizziness in comparison with placebo, and gout and muscle cramps in comparison with atenolol (MRC Working Party, 1992).

Thus, apart from the well-recognised adverse reactions associated with thiazide diuretics, such as gout, glucose intolerance and impotence, there is no evidence implicating this group of drugs as causing an impairment in global QOL.

Beta-blockers

Coope and Warrender (1986), using an extremely crude eight-symptom questionnaire which was mainly specific symptom orientated, failed to show an adverse effect of atenolol despite studying nearly 900 patients (Table 9.2). Unless they could not tolerate it, patients received 100 mg of atenolol, which is a higher dose than is necessary and would be likely to increase the risk of adverse reactions. The addition in some patients of bendrofluazide and methyldopa would also tend to increase adverse reactions in the treatment group. The failure to document adverse changes if only from methyldopa is probably a result of using a very short symptom checklist. The lack of any other QOL measures makes the study incapable of detecting any QOL effects, although the study achieved its primary aim of demonstrating cardiovascular benefit.

Goldstein *et al.* (1990) studied the effects on QOL in a group of nearly 700 men, who had passed their sixtieth birthday. Those who had not achieved an adequate response to hydrochlorothiazide alone were randomised to receive hydralazine, methyldopa, metoprolol or reserpine in addition. They found no differences in any tests, notably the modified CARE and the Zung Depression Scale.

As already discussed, the SHEP study employed atenolol as a second-line agent in patients not adequately controlled on chlorthalidone (SHEP Co-operative Research Group, 1991). The lack of difference in QOL measures between active treatment and control groups whilst predominantly reflecting the action of chlorthalidone does provide some evidence that atenolol does not have a detrimental effect as approximately 50% of patients received second-line therapy.

In a smaller study of 242 women with a mean age of 70 years no differences were seen between atenolol, enalapril and diltiazem (Applegate *et al.*, 1991).

The MRC trial of mild hypertension in older adults recruited patients with both isolated systolic and diastolic hypertension (MRC Working Party, 1992). Bird *et al.* (1990) reported no differences in cognitive function or Depression Questionnaire scores over the first 9 months of treatment in 2630 patients of both sexes taking atenolol 50 mg compared with a thiazide and placebo, no other QOL measures were included. Over the course of the study, however, there was a statistically significant excess of withdrawals in the atenolol group compared with placebo because of Raynaud's phenomenon, dyspnoea, nausea, dizziness, headache and bradycardia.

Using a placebo-controlled study of rather younger patients (from the age of 55 but with a mean of 66 years), McCorvey *et al.* (1993) compared hydrochlorothiazide, propranolol and enalapril. This study reported that the propranolol group performed significantly worse than the enalapril group on Part I of the Nottingham Health Profile (NHP). However, hypertensives were defined as having a history of hypertension with documented raised blood pressures within the previous year. In fact the mean diastolic blood pressure remained in the normotensive range (<90 mmHg) throughout the placebo phase, illustrating that the study group by definition was not hypertensive. In this setting it is not surprising that blood pressure was not significantly different between treatment groups and any QOL improvement that may be related to a blood pressure fall independent of direct drug effect could not be demonstrated.

The following year Croog *et al.* (1994) – the group who published the first major QOL study in hypertension – published their findings in a group of 309 elderly women given atenolol, enalapril and isradipine with or without hydrochlorothiazide. Other than the association of distress from cough associated with enalapril and dry mouth, associated with atenolol, no differences in QOL were seen.

In summary, there is little evidence of any effect on global QOL of beta-blockers, particularly the most widely used drug atenolol. There is, however, evidence linking beta-blockers generally, and atenolol in particular, with specific symptom adverse effects. Atenolol is not lipid soluble and would not be expected to penetrate the CNS unlike propranolol which, in addition to the negative effects reported by McCorvey *et al.* (1993) referred to above, was also found to produce deleterious effects on younger patients compared with captopril (Croog *et al.*, 1994).

Angiotensin-converting enzyme inhibitors

In a group of 24 elderly patients captopril was compared with bisoprolol. No differences were seen between active treatments or between placebo run-in and active treatments using four QOL questions at the end of a questionnaire (Bracchetti *et al.*, 1990). The power of the comparisons is uncertain.

Using a dose titration design, Applegate *et al.* (1991) compared enalapril with atenolol and diltiazem in 242 women with a mean age of 70. None of the QOL scores were significantly different between the treatments. When enalapril was compared in a small placebo-controlled study with propranolol, enalapril was significantly better than propranolol on an aggregated score derived from part I of the Nottingham Health Profile (McCorvey *et al.*, 1993). In a much larger study comparing captopril and enalapril in hypertensive women, an overall summary QOL score showed captopril to be better than enalapril (Testa *et al.*, 1993).

Calcium channel blockers

Only two reports have included a calcium channel blocker. Neither Skinner *et al.* (1992), who used nifedipine, nor Croog *et al.* (1994), who used isradipine, found any effects on QOL.

Other drugs

There are no data at present concerning the effects of other classes of drug on QOL in elderly patients with hypertension, although many of the older drugs have been used as additional therapy in patients not controlled, or not tolerating, first-time treatment. In younger patients, however, methyldopa has been shown to cause adverse QOL effects (Croog *et al.*, 1986). There is no data of any sort on the new classes of antihypertensives such as potassium channel blockers and angiotensin II receptor blockers.

Conclusions

A meta-analysis of all studies of QOL in hypertension up to 1990, including data on 1620 patients from nine published studies, identified a small beneficial effect of treatment on sleep, general well-being and mood but no such effect for sexual function (Beto and Bansal, 1992). When effects of individual classes of drugs were investigated, significant beneficial effects were confined to general well-being and mood with beta-blockers and diuretics having a significant effect on mood but only ACE inhibitors significantly improving well-being. This meta-analysis included only one study of older patients (Goldstein *et al.*, 1990), which itself did not show benefit. Thus, although it would seem likely that treating hypertension would confer quality of life benefit on elderly patients, there is as yet no evidence for such an effect. This is in contrast to the data on PP where there is evidence of benefit. The small number of placebo-controlled studies in elderly patients do provide some evidence that treatment does not result in a detrimental effect.

OTHER ADVERSE REACTIONS

While many drug-specific adverse reactions are widely appreciated, their true prevalence in elderly patients taking them on a long-term basis can only be assessed from large, placebo-controlled studies. This review, therefore, will cover the major intervention studies and will not include data on calcium antagonists and ACE inhibitors as they have not been the subject of studies so far reported, although such studies are underway (Dahlof *et al.*, 1993). Specific adverse effects for individual drugs are reviewed in Chapter 5.

Although the Hypertension, Detection and Follow-up Program (HDFP) compared two approaches to managing hypertension and cannot therefore yield data on drug-specific adverse reactions, it is interesting to note that for all adverse events the rate was lowest for the oldest group (age 60–69) than for any other age group (Curb *et al.*, 1988).

The European Working Party on High Blood Pressure in the Elderly (EWPHE) demonstrated that the treatment of hypertensive patients aged over 60 would, in return for the benefit of a reduction in cardiovascular endpoints, cause a significant number of ADRs (Fletcher *et al.*, 1991). An excess over placebo was seen of four cases of gout, 23 of raised creatinine, nine cases of diabetes mellitus, 124 with a dry mouth, 71 with diarrhoea and 71 with a serum potassium falling below 3.5 mmol/L per 1000 patient years. Diarrhoea and dry mouth were predominantly seen in patients who needed methyldopa as second-line treatment. Significant changes due to the first-line therapy – triamterene 50 mg and hydrochlorothiazide 25 mg – are summarised in Table 9.3.

Table 9.3 Rates per 1000 patient-years of statistically significant adverse events to active treatment (triamterene 50 mg and hydrochlorothiazide 25 mg with or without methyldopa) versus placebo in the European Working Party on High blood pressure in the Elderly (EWPHE) study

	Active	*Placebo*
Hyperuricaemia (men > 0.52 μmol/L; women > 0.46 μmol/L)	79.3	12.7
Gout	5.1	0.8
Raised creatinine (≥ 180 μmol/L)	33.3	9.8
Hypokalaemia (< 3.5 μmol/L) .	115.8	45.1

Second-line treatment with methyldopa was also associated with dry mouth and diarrhoea

The SHEP study, as a result of its much larger size, had substantial statistical power and was able to identify a range of adverse events occurring more frequently in patients receiving active treatment (thiazide and beta-blocker) than placebo (Table 9.4) (SHEP Co-operative Research Group, 1991). Although one or two of these significant differences might have occurred by chance, there were no symptoms that occurred significantly more frequently in the placebo group. It is of interest that although the prevalence of any specified problem ever classified as troublesome was very high, the difference between the groups was small. The SHEP study also documented the well-known but small changes in serum potassium, glucose, uric acid and cholesterol (Table 9.5).

Table 9.4   Prevalence of symptoms ever classified as troublesome or intolerable occurring significantly more commonly amongst patients taking active treatment versus those taking placebo in the Systolic Hypertension in the Elderly Program

	Prevalence %	
Symptom	*Active*	*Placebo*
Faintness on standing	12.8	10.6
Loss of consciousness/passing out	2.2	1.3
Heart beating unusually slowly	3.8	2.1
Chest pain or heaviness	28.0	21.3
Cold or numb hands	13.6	9.8
Ankle swelling	19.5	15.6
Trouble with memory/concentration	26.4	20.4
Problems with sexual function	4.8	3.2
Falls	12.8	10.4
Change in bowel habits	15.4	11.4
Excessive thirst	7.9	6.4
Skin rash or bruising	12.5	10.6
Unusual joint pain	36.4	31.4
Waking frequently at night to urinate	14.4	12.4
Any specified problem	91.8	86.4
Any specified problem characterised as intolerable	28.1	20.8

Table 9.5   Significant differences in serum biochemistry amongst patients taking active treatment (chlorthalidone $\pm$ atenolol or reserpine) versus those taking placebo in the Systolic Hypertension in the Elderly Program

	Active	*Placebo*
K^+ mmol/L	4.1	4.4
Uric acid mmol/L	374.7	327.1
Glucose mmol/L	6.4	6.1
Cholesterol mmol/L	6.3	6.1
Na^+ mmol/L	138.9	139.6

The Swedish Trial in Old Patients with Hypertension (STOP-Hypertension) study randomised rather older patients (70–84 years) to a diuretic, three different beta-blockers and placebo (Dahlof *et al.*, 1991). As more than two-thirds of randomised patients took both a diuretic and a beta-blocker to achieve blood pressure control, adverse effect data cannot easily be related to specific drugs. Biochemical changes very similar to those found in SHEP were seen (Ekbom *et al.*, 1992). Amongst a list of 14 symptoms, atenolol produced significant changes versus placebo in three (dry mouth, cold hands or feet and slow heart rate). Pindolol and hydrochlorothiazide produced one each and metoprolol no significant changes. It is worth noting that pindolol, a beta-blocker with marked intrinsic sympathomimetic activity (partial agonist), caused a significant increase in muscle discomfort or cramp which has been described before.

Table 9.6   Rates per 1000 patient-years of statistically significant differences in adverse events in the MRC Treatment Trial of Hypertension in Older Adults

Adverse event	Drug type	

Hydrochlorothiazide (25 mg) and amiloride (2.5 mg) vs placebo

	Diuretic	*Placebo*
Hyperglycaemia	6.9	2.7
Skin disorders	3.9	1.1
Nausea	7.4	1.1
Dizziness	7.4	1.2
Gout	4.4	0.1
Muscle cramp	5.2	0.1

Atenolol (50 mg) vs placebo

	Beta-blocker	*Placebo*
Hyperglycaemia	5.8	2.7
Raynaud's phenomenon	11.3	0.3
Dyspnoea	22.9	1.1
Lethargy	19.1	2.0
Nausea	4.1	1.1
Dizziness	10.6	1.2
Headache	7.2	1.1
Bradycardia	28.0	0.0

Atenolol (50 mg) vs hydrochlorothiazide (25 mg) and amiloride (2.5 mg)

	Beta-blocker	*Diuretic*
Raynaud's phenomenon	11.3	0.6
Dyspnoea	22.9	0.8
Lethargy	19.1	4.1
Headache	7.2	2.5
Bradycardia	28.0	0.0
Gout	0	4.4
Muscle cramps	1.0	5.2

The Medical Research Council trial of treatment of hypertension in older adults reported twice as many withdrawals due to adverse events from the beta-blocker group as from the diuretic group (32/year diuretic; 66/year beta-blocker; 16/year placebo) (MRC Working Party, 1992). This study was similar in size to SHEP and was able to demonstrate a number of adverse events occurring more frequently in the diuretic and beta-blocker groups compared with patients taking placebo (Table 9.6). Apart from bradycardia, dyspnoea and lethargy during atenolol treatment, the incidence of individual adverse events was low with most occurring less frequently than 1 per 100 patients per year. In addition to the well-known associations such as gout and hyperglycaemia with the diuretic and bradycardia, dyspnoea, lethargy and Raynaud's phenomenon with the beta-blocker, less well-recognised associations were identified, such as skin reactions, dizziness, nausea and muscle cramps with hydrochlorothiazide and amiloride and nausea, dizziness and headache with atenolol (Table 9.6).

Conclusions

Traditional first-line therapy for hypertension in elderly patients – a low dose thiazide diuretic – is remarkably well tolerated but undoubtedly causes a small but definite excess over placebo of a range of symptoms and biochemical changes. Withdrawal rates due to ADRs are, not unexpectedly, also higher. The MRC and STOP-Hypertension studies also demonstrated that atenolol has an adverse effect profile that is, in general, less good than the thiazide comparator. Similar large-scale, long-term follow-up data is unavailable to date for the newer agents.

REFERENCES

Amery A, Birkenhager W, Brixko P et al. 1985. Mortality and morbidity results from the European Working Party on High Blood Pressure in the Elderly trial. *Lancet* i, 1349–54.

Applegate WB, Phillips HL, Schnaper H et al. 1991. A randomized controlled trial of the effects of three antihypertensive agents on blood pressure control and quality of life in older women. *Archives of Internal Medicine* **151**, 1817–23.

Applegate WB, Pressel S, Wittes J et al. 1994. Impact of the treatment of isolated systolic hypertension on behavioral variables. Results from the systolic hypertension in the elderly program. *Archives of Internal Medicine* **154**, 2154–60.

Bergner M, Bobbitt RA, Carter WB, Gilson BS 1981. The Sickness Impact Profile: Development and final revision of a health status measure. *Medical Care* **19**, 787–805.

Beto JA, Bansal VK 1992. Quality of life in treatment of hypertension. A metaanalysis of clinical trials. *American Journal of Hypertension* **5**, 125–33.

Bird AS, Blizard RA, Mann AH 1990. Treating hypertension in the older person: an evaluation of the association of blood pressure level and its reduction with cognitive performance. *Journal of Hypertension* **8**, 147–52.

Bowling A 1995. *Measuring disease*. Buckingham: Open University Press.

Bracchetti D, Gradnik R, Alberti A et al. 1990. A double blind comparison of bisoprolol and captopril for treatment of essential hypertension. *Cardiovascular Drug Therapy* **4**, 216–64.

Bulpitt CJ, Fletcher AE 1990a. The measurement of quality of life in hypertensive patients: a practical approach. *British Journal of Clinical Pharmacology* **30**, 355–64.

Bulpitt CJ, Fletcher AE 1990b. Drug treatment and quality of life in the elderly. *Clinics in Geriatric Medicine* **6**, 309–17.

Calman KC 1984. Quality of life in cancer patients – an hypothesis. *Journal of Medical Ethics* **10**, 124–7.

Coope J, Warrender TS 1986. Randomised trial of treatment of hypertension in elderly patients in primary care. *British Medical Journal* **293**, 1145–51.

Croog SH, Elias MF, Colton T *et al.* 1994. Effects of antihypertensive medications on quality of life in elderly hypertensive women. *American Journal of Hypertension* **7**, 329–39.

Croog SH, Levine S, Testa MA *et al.* 1986. The effects of antihypertensive therapy on the quality of life. *New England Journal of Medicine* **314**, 1657–64.

Curb JD, Schneider K, Taylor JO, Maxwell M, Shulman N 1988. Antihypertensive drug side effects in the Hypertension Detection and Follow-up Program. *Hypertension* **11**, 1151–5.

Dahlof B, Hansson L, Lindholm LH *et al.* 1993. STOP-Hypertension 2, a prospective intervention trial of 'newer' versus 'older' treatment alternatives in old patients with hypertension. Swedish Trial in Old Patients with Hypertension. *Blood Pressure* **2**, 136–41.

Dahlof B, Lindholm LH, Hansson L, Schersten B, Ekbom T, Wester P-O 1991. Morbidity and mortality in the Swedish Trial in Old Patients with Hypertension (STOP-Hypertension). *Lancet* **338**, 1281–5.

Ekbom T, Dahlof B, Hansson L, Lindholm LH, Schersten B, Wester PO 1992. Antihypertensive efficacy and side effects of three β blockers and a diuretic in elderly hypertensives: a report from the STOP-Hypertension study. *Journal of Hypertension* **10**, 1525–30.

Farmer ME, Kittner SJ, Abbott RD, Wolz MM, Wolf PA, White LR 1990. Longitudinally measured blood pressure, antihypertensive medication use, and cognitive performance: the Framingham Study. *Journal of Clinical Epidemiology* **43**, 475–80.

Farmer ME, White LR, Abbott RD *et al.* 1987. Blood pressure and cognitive performance. *American Journal of Epidemiology* **126**, 1103–14.

Fletcher A, Amery A, Birkenhager W *et al.* 1991. Risks and benefits in the trial of the European Working Party on High Blood Pressure in the Elderly. *Journal of Hypertension* **9**, 225–30.

Gengo FM, Fagan SC, de Padova A, Miller JK, Kinkel PR 1988. The effect of beta-blockers on mental performance on older hypertensive patients. *Archives of Internal Medicine* **148**, 779–84.

Goldstein G, Materson BJ, Cushman WC *et al.* 1990. Treatment of hypertension in the elderly: II. Cognitive and behavioral function. Results of a Department of Veterans Affairs Cooperative Study. *Hypertension* **15**, 361–9.

Gurland JG, Teresi J, Smith WM, Black D, Hughes G, Edlavitch S 1988. Effects of treatment for isolated systolic hypertension on cognitive status and depression in the elderly. *Journal of the American Geriatric Society* **36**, 1015–22.

Hamilton M, Thompson EN, Wisniewski TKM 1964. The role of blood pressure control in preventing complications of hypertension. *Lancet* **i**, 235–8.

Hunt SM 1984. Nottingham health profile. In Lenger NK, Mattson ME, Farberg CP, Elinson J (eds) *Assessment of quality of life in clinical trials of cardiovascular therapy*. New York: Le Jacq.

Hypertension Detection and Follow up Program Co-operative Group 1979. Five-year findings of the hypertension detection and follow-up program. I. Reduction in mortality of persons with high blood pressure, including mild hypertension. Hypertension Detection and Follow-up Program Co-operative Group. *Journal of the American Medical Association* **242**, 2562–71.

Kalra L, Jackson SHD, Swift CG 1993a. Effect of antihypertensive treatment on psychomotor performance in the elderly. *Journal of Human Hypertension* **7**, 285–90.

Kalra L, Jackson SHD, Swift CG 1993b. Psychomotor performance in elderly hypertensive patients. *Journal of Human Hypertension* **7**, 279–84.

Kalra L, Swift CG, Jackson SHD 1994. Psychomotor performance and antihypertensive treatment. *British Journal of Clinical Pharmacology* **37**, 165–72.

Kostis JB, Rosen RC, Holzer BC, Randolph C, Taska LS, Miller MH 1990. CNS side effects of centrally-active antihypertensive agents: a prospective, placebo-controlled study of sleep, mood state, and cognitive and sexual function in hypertensive males. *Psychopharmacology* **102**, 163–70.

McCorvey E Jr, Wright JT Jr, Culbert JP, McKenney JM, Proctor JD, Annett MP 1993. Effect of hydrochlorothiazide, enalapril, and propranolol on quality of life and cognitive and motor function in hypertensive patients. *Clinical Pharmacology* **12**, 300–5.

MRC Working Party 1992. Medical Research Council trial of treatment of hypertension in older adults: principal results. *British Medical Journal* **304**, 405–12.

Shapiro AP, Nixon P, Miller RE, Manuck SB, Jennings R, King HE 1989. Behavioural consequences of hypertension: effects of age and type of antihypertensive agent. *Journal of Human Hypertension* **3**, 435–42.

SHEP Co-operative Research Group 1991. Prevention of stroke by antihypertensive drug treatment in older persons with isolated systolic hypertension. Final results of the Systolic Hypertension in the Elderly Program (SHEP). SHEP Co-operative Research Group. *Journal of the American Medical Association* **265**, 3255–64.

Skinner MH, Futterman A, Morrissette D, Thompson LW, Hoffman BB, Blaschke TF 1992. Atenolol compared with nifedipine: effect on cognitive function and mood in elderly hypertensive patients. *Annals of Internal Medicine* **116**, 615–23.

Solomen S, Hotchkiss E, Saravay SM, Bayer C, Ramsay P 1983. Impairment of memory function by antihypertensive medication. *Archives of General Psychology* **40**, 1109–12.

Testa MA, Anderson RB, Nackley JF, Hollenberg NK 1993. Quality of life and antihypertensive therapy in men. A comparison of captopril with enalapril. The Quality-of-Life Hypertension Study Group. *New England Journal of Medicine* **328**, 907–13.

Wallace R, Lemke JH, Morris MC 1985. Relationship of free recall memory to hypertension in the elderly: The Iowa 65+ rural health study. *Journal of Chronic Disease* **38**, 475–81.

Wurzelmann J, Frishman WH, Aronson M, Masur D, Ooi WL 1987. Neuropsychological effects of antihypertensive drugs. *Cardiology Clinics* **5**, 689–701.

CHAPTER 10

Overview

ANDREW K SCOTT ————————————————————————————

INTRODUCTION

When we decide that elderly patients should be offered treatment for hypertension, most accept our decision with little comment. If questions are asked, they are usually related to the need for treatment and whether or not it will do any good. For example:

1. Do I really have high blood pressure when I feel so well?
2. Will treatment do any good at my age?
3. Is this the best treatment available, my friend is taking . . . .?
4. Do the tablets have any side effects?

In this final chapter, I propose to try to provide answers to these questions on the basis of information contained within the book. I shall also consider how treatment can be delivered in a cost-effective manner to all elderly people who need it. Appropriate management of a common problem like hypertension should be available to all and not depend on the presence of a local specialist clinic or individual doctor with an interest in the subject.

The aim of treating hypertension is to self-evidently prevent the consequences of the high blood pressure. By far the most common problems are heart disease and stroke. Any intervention needs to be effective in reducing these problems or it will not be worthwhile either for the individual patient or the health service. Many of the consequences of hypertension appear to be related to the severity and duration of hypertension as discussed in Chapter 3. However, we still do not know whether or not all agents that lower blood pressure will be effective in reducing the important clinical complications. The level of blood pressure at which to start treatment is very important but easier to define in population terms than for an individual patient.

DO I HAVE HIGH BLOOD PRESSURE?

Since there is no clear cut-off between a blood pressure which does no harm and one that increases the risk of vascular disease, the level of blood pressure we choose to define 'hypertension' will always be arbitrary. When patients ask if they have high blood pressure we need to consider both the level of blood pressure and whether or not it is sustained. Most patients are happy to accept that there is an uncertain area when blood pressures are borderline and require observation rather than early treatment, albeit as part of a holistic approach taking account of other risk factors. This will be considered in more detail later. Although there is some disagreement about the level of blood pressure at which treatment should be started, the differences are relatively small and probably not a major factor in determining the need for, and success of, treatment.

Two of the main ways of ensuring that resources used to treat hypertension are directed to those most likely to benefit are screening combined with steps taken to ensure an accurate diagnosis of sustained hypertension. Clearly, the only method for detection of all hypertension in a population is to screen the entire population. However, such an approach can cause problems. Patients found to have a raised pressure on their screening visit but who are subsequently found to be normal will have been caused unnecessary worry. Many patients will also be labelled hypertensive, though they do not have true sustained hypertension, as discussed below. There is good evidence of ill health caused by screening programmes and these can only be justified if there is no other method and the end results outweigh the adverse effects. In addition, such a widespread programme would be expensive and need to be repeated every few years. On the other hand, the problem cannot simply be ignored. In many countries an intermediate approach has been adopted.

For example, in Norway (and the United Kingdom) almost all (about 90%) of the adult population attend their general practitioner over a 5-year period (Holmen *et al.*, 1991). This presents the possibility of opportunistic screening. If the blood pressure is measured during a routine consultation there is likely to be less stress on the patient. Many general practices have adopted this approach and developed systems for marking the patient record folders to remind the doctor that blood pressure needs to be measured. In addition, all patients over the age of 75 years in the UK are required to be offered a general screen, which includes blood pressure measurement. Some patients will be missed by such an approach but, since the numbers are relatively small, a more extensive type of screening cannot be justified either in terms of extra benefit over risks or the costs involved. If all practices were to adopt this approach then the proportion of hypertensive patients in the population known to their doctor should rise from the present level of around 50% to 90%. This figure could be even higher in elderly patients because they are more likely to attend their doctor within a given time.

Whatever method is used to detect hypertension, it is still necessary to act on the blood pressure reading, in particular to decide whether treatment is necessary. This is one of the most difficult aspects of management, and one in which errors are often made. Even in a clinical trial, a high percentage (perhaps 20–50%) of patients are found to develop normal blood pressure when they are randomised to the placebo arm of the trial. Ambulatory blood pressure monitoring studies and studies of withdrawal of medication also suggest that up to 50% of patients labelled as having mild to moderate hypertension do not have a sustained rise in blood pressure.

The level of risk of patients with labile blood pressure is not known. Since treated blood pressure appears to be a better guide to prognosis than initial blood pressure then these patients should be at low risk if the pressure settles.

However, their risk may be higher than for patients who have normal blood pressure on screening. There is no evidence as to whether or not treatment helps such patients.

Before answering the patient's question 'Do I really have high blood pressure?', reasonable steps must be taken to establish an accurate diagnosis. The gold standard at present would appear to be 24-hour ambulatory monitoring using a validated fully automatic system. This could not be achieved for all patients with present resources. Careful selection of patients using existing guidelines would greatly reduce the numbers requiring 24-hour monitoring. Ambulatory recordings should be obtained for all borderline or doubtful cases and for those with relatively 'mild' hypertension. Clearly, if blood pressure settles with time, 24-hour monitoring is not required. The higher the level of blood pressure, the lower the chance of a false positive diagnosis. In my experience, failure to respond to multiple drug therapy (assuming compliance has been confirmed) also points to the possibility of white-coat hypertension but care must be taken not to miss an underlying cause of secondary hypertension.

WILL TREATMENT DO ANY GOOD AT MY AGE?

This is perhaps the easiest question to answer if the patient is under 80 years old but more difficult in the over 85 age group. If a thiazide diuretic is used as first-line treatment in a patient under 80, we can confidently state that the risk of stroke will be reduced by about a third and that of heart disease by around a fifth. We can also explain that the benefits are clearer in patients aged 60–80 years than in younger age groups and talk about the number of patient-years of treatment required to avoid one adverse event. Beta-blockers can also be claimed to have some benefit but less marked than for thiazide diuretics. At present it is not possible to give an accurate estimate of benefit for newer agents.

For patients over the age of 85 years the question is more difficult. Relatively few patients over this age have been included in studies published to date. Some evidence of the benefit of lowering blood pressure needs to be balanced against studies that show better survival in patients with higher blood pressure. Studies currently under way should give a definitive answer to this problem, but perhaps not for several more years.

IS THIS THE BEST TREATMENT?

There is a natural feeling by some patients that newer, more expensive treatments must be better. This is especially so if a friend has just been started on a new agent that has been highly praised by the doctor and which has effectively reduced the blood pressure. After a full explanation, most patients seem happy to accept low dose thiazide diuretics on the basis of proven efficacy in stroke prevention and low risk of adverse effects. The 'old age' of these drugs should be seen as a major advantage since it is unlikely that any serious adverse events are waiting to be discovered. With newer agents there is always a risk of serious toxicity occurring in a small percentage of patients but not being discovered until the drug has been used for several years. The cloud hanging over short-acting calcium antagonists as discussed in Chapters 4 and 5 should serve as a reminder that good evidence-based medicine is often ignored in the face of aggressive pharmaceutical marketing based on intermediate endpoints rather than morbidity and mortality. (See also Appendix.)

If the patient also suffers from cardiac failure, angiotensin-converting enzyme inhibitors (ACE inhibitors) can at least be supported as treatment for the failure though we still do not know if these drugs prevent stroke. Loop diuretics are usually used in combination with ACE inhibitors in the treatment of cardiac failure. In hypertensive patients with failure it might be better to combine a thiazide with the ACE inhibitor. A larger dose of thiazide would, of course, be necessary to achieve adequate diuresis. Again, however, there is no evidence to clarify whether or not such an approach is better than loop diuretic plus ACE inhibitor.

ADVERSE EFFECTS

As in many areas of medicine it is difficult to know how much to tell each patient. Clearly, patients have a right to know about all the side effects if they so wish. However, for most patients it seems more reasonable to discuss only the more common adverse effects unless the patient specifically asks for further information.

How common is 'common'? Problems with an incidence of 10% or more certainly need to be discussed; for example, cough with ACE inhibitors or flushing with calcium channel antagonists. Rare events with a risk of less than one in a thousand do not need to be routinely mentioned; for example, blood dyscrasias with any drug. Serious effects warrant mention more than minor ones with the same frequency. Where should the line be drawn? There is a wide range of opinions on how much to tell patients and few studies have looked at how much patients are told and how much they want to know. I am unaware of any study which has investigated this in the treatment of hypertension in elderly patients. It would appear, anecdotally, that we are inconsistent in what we tell patients in relation to the relative risks of adverse effects and also in the advice we give at different times.

Should we, for example, mention renal failure with ACE inhibitors (approximate risk 1 in 100); angio-edema with ACE inhibitors (risk 1 in 1000); cardiac failure with calcium channel antagonists (risk varies with different drugs); bronchospasm with beta-blockers (risk 1 in 50 in non-asthmatics); rash with thiazides (1 in 100); impotence with thiazides (1 in 50) or other agents; diabetes with thiazides (risk very low with low dose)? There is no easy answer and to explain several potential problems takes time. In a move to try to increase patient awareness of the drugs they are taking and their potential adverse effects some clinics have produced patient information leaflets. There appears to be some benefit from such an approach, at least in the short term.

Although most patients appear to benefit from having more information in a form they can understand, there are exceptions. Some patients become very preoccupied by adverse effects that they have been told about or read in the patient information leaflet. In extreme examples, it becomes very difficult to give effective treatment, with problems occurring with all the drugs prescribed. Eventually it may become necessary to strike a bargain with the patient about what is acceptable. This requires a detailed explanation of the risks of untreated hypertension and the likely time course of side effects (real or imagined) if drug treatment continues. Fortunately such patients are rare and it is essential to avoid too negative an approach. Many adverse effects become less troublesome with time if patients can be encouraged to continue with treatment; for example, flushing with calcium antagonists. However, only the patient can decide if the discomfort of taking medication is worth 'learning to live with' when set against the likely benefits of treatment.

In treating hypertension we need to consider the needs of the patient, the deliverers of health care and the health service. While the overall aims are hopefully similar for each group, there are obviously differences in priorities. Little research is carried out on this aspect of medical practice. Much remains to be done before we have the means to deliver ideal treatment for hypertension.

WHAT DO HYPERTENSIVE PATIENTS NEED FROM HEALTH SERVICES?

The first choice of patients would be to have treatment that cures rather than controls. A short course of a drug to reverse the underlying deficit in the way an antibiotic cures infection is expected by many patients. Despite explanations to the contrary, some stop their medication when the blood pressure falls to normal levels. Clearly there is still a need for research into the cause of hypertension with the hope that a mechanism can be found to reverse the underlying problem on a permanent basis.

For the foreseeable future we are faced with trying to achieve optimum control over many years of treatment. Patients generally want a treatment that is going to be effective, has no side effects, is simple to take and is part of a holistic approach to their care. There is room for improvement in all of these areas.

The main groups of antihypertensive drugs show similar levels of efficacy, but, generally, the fall in blood pressure is relatively small such that about 50% of patients require two or more drugs. It would be useful to have a more powerful drug available, providing there was no increase in adverse effects. However, the main research effort must be in establishing which drugs are most effective at reducing complications. It is clear that the risk of stroke can be reduced by around 30% using a thiazide diuretic based regime. This is of the order of the increase in stroke risk due to hypertension. It is thus unlikely that other drugs will improve on this response unless they have other properties that reverse other factors affecting stroke risk. We should have some answers to this question by the end of the century when ongoing clinical trials have been completed. However, the situation with regard to ischaemic heart disease is less clear and, in theory, other drugs might be better than thiazides. It is regrettable that studies looking at the effect of other drug groups were not started at an earlier time.

It is unlikely that any powerful drug would be free of adverse effects. It would therefore be helpful if there was some way of predicting which patients are at risk from a particular drug group. For a small number of adverse effects this is possible. For example, patients with cardiomegaly are more likely to develop cardiac failure if given a beta-blocker; patients with peripheral vascular disease are more likely to have renal artery stenosis and develop renal failure on ACE inhibitors. Particular effort needs to be concentrated on avoiding the serious adverse effects.

Simplicity of drug regimen with minimal disruption of lifestyle is essential for most patients. The ideal drug in this respect is a long-acting one that can be taken once daily at a time convenient to the patient. We obviously already have drugs of this type in each group; for example, all thiazides, atenolol, amlodipine and lisinopril. This is important for patients with active lives. Most elderly patients are active and appreciate not having to carry bottles of tablets with them when they go out. Once-daily dosing is also of benefit in patients with memory problems. It is easier for carers to supervise medication on a once-daily basis. Also if dosing boxes are used it is easier to keep the number of tablets to a minimum.

Lifestyle changes are more difficult. Changes that cause major disruption are unlikely to be adopted by elderly patients. Changes made should be capable of fitting easily into the patient's life. Exercise should take the form of walking for most patients since cycling or swimming are not suitable for those who have not been on a bicycle for 50 years or have no nearby pool. Dietary changes, similarly, should be selected to achieve benefit by fitting the patient's needs, though encouraging a move away from the most hazardous elements such as very high saturated fat or salt intake.

There is great enthusiasm at present for a holistic approach to care but this may be difficult when time is limited. Few would argue with the need for a holistic approach to the management of hypertension, dealing with factors that increase blood pressure as well as those which increase the risk of vascular disease in other ways. As discussed above, lowering of blood pressure alone will achieve only a 30% reduction in stroke and, on present knowledge, 20% in heart disease. Further reduction in these complications requires effective action on other risk factors. We already know what most of these are but further research needs to address the optimum ways of implementing strategies to reduce the risks. Obvious examples are smoking cessation, weight reduction, moderating excessive alcohol intake and increasing exercise. Psychological factors have received attention with attempts to control blood pressure by relaxation therapy or meditation.

An interesting group is patients with labile/white-coat hypertension. What is it in these patients that maintains a high level of blood pressure in the clinic while others settle after the first few visits? Better understanding of the mechanisms for continuing high clinic pressures in a significant proportion of patients might lead to the development of strategies to minimise this problem. There may be factors in the clinic, rather than the patient, contributing to this problem, and they may therefore be more amenable to change. Long waits to be seen, stressful surroundings and poor attitude of staff are unacceptable. We may be unaware of what our style of medical practice does to the patient's blood pressure. In the Aberdeen blood pressure clinic a study was conducted of the effects of five different doctors on blood pressure measurement. Semi-automatic sphygmomanometers were used to avoid observer variation in the actual pressure measurement. Clear differences were observed between different doctors (Jamieson *et al.*, unpublished results). Further research in this area would be valuable.

A decision to treat should consider the risk of vascular disease for the individual patient, taking all potential risk factors into account. This has been calculated for various cholesterol concentrations in the presence of the four other main risk factors – hypertension, smoking, diabetes, left ventricular hypertrophy (Haq *et al.*, 1995). Other authors have suggested a similar approach. For example, a report of the New Zealand National Advisory Committee on Core Health and Disability Services on the management of hypertension recommended that 'decisions to treat raised blood pressure should be based primarily on the estimated absolute risk of cardiovascular disease rather than on blood pressure alone' (Jackson *et al.*, 1993). As an example, they point out that if treatment is based on blood pressure alone, guidelines suggest that a 60-year-old woman with a diastolic pressure of 100 mmHg and no other risk factors would be treated, whereas a 70-year-old man with diastolic pressure of 95 mmHg and multiple cardiovascular risk factors would not be treated. This is despite the fact that the 60-year-old woman has only a 10% risk of a cardiovascular event over the next 10 years, whereas the 70-year-old man has a 50% chance. Treatment of blood pressure would reduce the risk to 7% for the 60-year-old woman and 33% for the 70-year-old man. The New Zealand report suggests that treatment for mild hypertension (150–170/90–100 mmHg) should be given only if there is a 20% or greater chance of a major cardiovascular event over the next 10 years. At this level of risk, 150 people would need to be treated to prevent one cardiovascular event per year. Important risk factors in this context are age, cigarette smoking, high total cholesterol or low high-density lipoprotein or both, diabetes, male sex and a family history of premature coronary heart disease. All elderly (over 70 years) men meeting the blood pressure criteria should be treated. They also suggest that all elderly women should be treated if blood pressure is greater than 170/100 or if blood pressure is greater than 150/90 with one or more other risk factors.

While there is room for debate about the cut-off figures, the general principles seem correct. Most elderly patients clearly justify treatment when an accurate diagnosis of sustained hypertension is made. Discussion should concentrate on not wasting resources on younger patients with low risk of a cardiovascular event. In financial terms, for a diastolic blood pressure of 95–99 mmHg, it costs £55 000 per additional life-year gained for a 40-year-old man compared with £5600 for a 60-year-old woman and £300 for a 70-year-old man (Swales, 1995). These costs are for treating the hypertension and clearly do not take into account all the costs of hypertension to the community and the benefits of avoiding complications.

WHAT DO DELIVERERS OF CARE NEED?

In many respects we require the same as our patients. An effective, safe treatment which is simple to administer certainly provides for an easier working life! Hypertension is such a common problem that it cannot be left to specialists in that field. All staff directly involved in patient care should be reasonably familiar with the condition. Hypertension tends to be seen as an 'easy' disorder by many doctors who simply measure blood pressure, start treatment and hope for the best. However, much published research and many local audits have confirmed that the management of hypertension is far from ideal. Earlier chapters have shown that there are many problems related to both diagnosis and treatment.

Blood pressure measurement is difficult to perform with accuracy unless great care is taken. Standards of measurement are not high. False positive diagnosis is common. Patients who should be treated are not, or only partly, treated. Follow-up is haphazard. Drug choice is often irrational with little sign of evidence-based practice. In a local audit conducted in 1993, results similar to national trends were found (Roomi and Scott, unpublished data). Working backwards from those listed before 1992 on a computerised database in two hospitals, 100 patients with hypertension were identified. The diagnosis of hypertension was not properly established in 77% of patients. Digit preference was rife with only 5% of readings being made to the nearest 2 mmHg. Choice of drug was inappropriate for many patients. Control was good in only 51% with little attempt made to achieve better control or to document that this was the best possible for the individual patient.

It is unrealistic to expect all practitioners to have detailed knowledge of all diseases but they do need to know where to get information when their expertise is limited. As a result, several sets of guidelines have been produced on the management of hypertension. They are in broad agreement, though there are some differences in the recommended level at which to start treatment and in the choice of first-line drug. Unfortunately, the production of guidelines does not ensure that these are followed unless there is a good clinical reason for deviation. The guidelines tend to be aimed at hypertension in the general adult population though some advice is usually included on elderly patients.

Guidelines need to define when to treat, how to treat and the target blood pressure. Clearly, severe and accelerated hypertension require early treatment but most patients seen have mild to moderate hypertension. All the guidelines recommend an initial period of observation before starting drug treatment. This is 3–6 months in most guidelines (Sever *et al.*, 1993; JNC on Detection, Evaluation and Treatment of High Blood Pressure, 1993) but the Australian guidelines suggest 1 month (Hypertension Guidelines Committee, 1991). Non-pharmacological measures may be tried during this time. The suggested blood pressure at which treatment should be started after the period of observation ranges from 90–100 mmHg diastolic and 140–170 mmHg systolic. On balance a diastolic of 95–100 and systolic of 160 seem to have most support. All agree that the threshold for treatment should be lowered in the presence of other cardiovascular risk factors. The New Zealand guidelines give more detailed advice on when to treat in the presence of other risk factors as discussed above.

The question of how to treat has been most debated in recent years. Several guidelines opted for diuretics or beta-blockers as first-line treatment but others have allowed use of all drug groups. The British Hypertension Society initially opted for diuretic/beta-blocker but later the committee was divided, with some members opting for newer drug classes. Time will tell if they are correct but at present there is little evidence to suggest anything other than thiazide diuretic for first-line treatment of elderly hypertensive patients unless there are specific reasons for avoiding this group of drugs. Evidence in terms of proven efficacy, low toxicity and very low costs are very much in favour of low dose thiazide diuretics.

Target blood pressure is generally set at less than 140/90, though the British Hypertension Society suggests a systolic of less than 160 mmHg. Debate on whether lower pressures should be aimed at has focused on a possible increase in risk of coronary death if blood pressure is too low. The Hypertension Optimal Treatment study may well provide answers to this question.

Elderly patients have received relatively little separate consideration in these guidelines. The World Health Organisation guidelines point out the potential for greater benefits in older patients and use the same suggested level as for younger adults at which to start treatment (160/95 mmHg). The British Hypertension Society, on the other hand, suggests that elderly patients aged 60–80 years should be treated at 160/90 mmHg compared with a diastolic pressure of 100 in younger patients (unless there is target organ damage). They also recommend that for patients over 80 years there is little evidence to support benefit from initiating treatment.

Our target must be to move as far away from the rule of halves as possible with better detection, initiation of treatment and control of blood pressure. A recent study from the Newcastle area suggests that some progress is being made, with about 70% of people with raised blood pressure detected and 74% of those detected on treatment, though only 53% of treated patients were adequately controlled (Ford *et al.*, 1996). Is it unreasonable to aim for detection of hypertension in at least 90% of the elderly population; to treat all of those who need therapy and want it; and to achieve good control in at least 90% of patients on long-term follow-up? All of this could be achieved with delivery of an efficient service designed for the needs of the patient and the practitioner.

WHAT DOES THE HEALTH SERVICE NEED?

Again the needs must encompass those of the patient and of the practitioners as discussed above. However, health services have other considerations that may be given less weight by doctors and patients. Whether health care is funded by taxation, and free at the point of delivery, or directly by the patient through private funding/insurance or somewhere between the extremes, cost is important. No health system has unlimited funding and choices need to be made to obtain the best overall value for money. The economics of managing hypertension were covered in Chapter 8 and it is clear that much more research is required.

Within hypertension, as in other fields, it seems sensible to target resources to those most likely to benefit. The health service needs information on the relative risks of individuals such that a decision can be made on when to start treatment. For example, a 40-year-old man with a slightly raised blood pressure and no other risk factors has a low risk of a vascular event in the next 10 years. Many hundreds of patient-years of treatment would be necessary to prevent one vascular event. Many such patients are treated but the money could be better spent elsewhere. Elderly patients are at higher individual risk for the same level of blood pressure and a good economic case can be made for spending resources on this age group. As discussed in Chapter 8, it is essential that the correct type of evaluation is carried out so that all relevant factors (all direct costs, outcome, costs of failure of prevention, etc.) are taken into consideration. Too little emphasis is put on treating hypertension in elderly patients. The financial benefits of doing so, in addition to the benefits to the patient, need to be clearly determined if we are to defend the needs of this group.

Given that there is little to choose between the different drug classes in terms of blood pressure reduction, any study using blood pressure as an endpoint will show that the cheapest drug is the most cost-effective unless it has large monitoring costs. Even allowing for plasma electrolyte concentration measurement costs, low dose thiazide diuretics work out cheapest. In the UK, the drug cost of low dose generic bendrofluazide is, remarkably, under £2.00 per year. On that basis, many thousands of pounds are wasted every year in each region where other drugs are used first. The extra expense can only be justified if there is extra benefit in terms of reduction of real endpoints such as stroke or heart disease. Unfortunately this information is not yet available to purchasers of health care. As discussed above, it is unlikely that there will be better reduction in stroke risk with newer hypotensive drugs but there might be in cardiac risk. Time will tell!

One difficulty in discussing relative drug costs is that good information relating to routine clinical practice is not readily available. Most drug cost comparisons simply take the recommended dose range and compare costs at the upper and lower limits. This may be very misleading as good data on relative efficacy is often unavailable. Also drug use in practice may differ from that in clinical trials. A wide variety of ACE inhibitors is now available and a major marketing claim for some drugs is on the grounds of cost compared with other agents. Ramipril was claimed to be cheaper than enalapril or captopril. However, in a comparison of actual costs of these drugs in routine practice in 100 hypertensive patients, enalapril was found to be cheaper than ramipril for a similar level of blood pressure control (Roomi and Scott, unpublished data). Enalapril seemed to offer control of blood pressure at doses below the maximum suggested, whereas many patients required full doses of ramipril. This study also showed the excessive costs when once-daily drugs were prescribed two or three times daily. There is often little difference in price between different doses of a drug, therefore giving a single 10 mg tablet costs less than 5 mg twice daily. Clearly the number of patients in this study was small and further work is required to produce robust information.

Non-pharmacological treatment costs are also considered in Chapter 8. As was seen, these are relatively expensive since they involve much staff time initially. The poor response of blood pressure to such measures compared to drug treatment was covered in Chapter 7. The effect of non-pharmacological treatments on vascular endpoints is not yet established. In terms of funding it does not seem justified to divert resources to non-pharmacological methods as a sole treatment for hypertension. In routine practice non-pharmacological measures are usually suggested in addition to drug treatment as part of overall management. Non-pharmacological treatment should be considered both in terms of the effect on blood pressure and the effect on other risk factors. More research is required in this area to allow purchasers and prescribers to make more rational decisions.

Health services also require good quality audit data to ensure that the needs of the population for which they are responsible are being met.

HOW SHOULD SERVICES TO TREAT HYPERTENSION BE DELIVERED?

The bulk of treatment for a common problem such as hypertension must be delivered through community services with a lesser role for hospital specialists. In the UK the general practitioner acts as a gatekeeper and decides who to refer to hospital. There is wide variation in referral rates depending on the skills and experience of individual GPs and whether or not there is a specialist with an interest in hypertension in the local hospital. A system whereby neither GP nor hospital doctor has a special interest in hypertension will never achieve the results required on a population basis. The ideal service should provide prompt, accurate diagnosis followed by effective treatment where indicated and a safe follow-up procedure. Some general practitioners have set up hypertension clinics for their practice and have purchased ambulatory blood pressure monitors to improve diagnosis. Such practitioners may refer only their difficult hypertensive patients to hospital for follow-up and treatment. Follow-up can be organised by the practice computer with a system that identifies defaulters and ensures that a further appointment is arranged. The traditional type of general practice and hospital follow-up system allows too many patients to be lost to follow-up by default.

While most patients must be dealt with in the community, there is a place for the hospital specialist and good links are required between them. Hypertension is a condition highly appropriate for shared care. While there are some shared-care systems in operation, the published literature is sparse. In the Grampian Region of the UK the Aberdeen-based computer assisted shared-care system, was well received by local practitioners with 82% of 1426 patients under general practice follow-up (Petrie *et al.*, 1985). The scheme aims to facilitate the exchange of clinically important information between hospital and general practice and to achieve target levels of blood pressure with treatment in patients at highest risk of cardiovascular events. Patients move between hospital and general practice as necessary with the less well controlled patients being concentrated under hospital follow-up. At the most recent visit prior to publication in 1985, 32% of patients in the hospital aspect and 10% in the general practice aspect had blood pressure records above target. Shared care for hypertension was set up in Glasgow in 1985 and has improved patient care with a streamlined organisation of service (Hannah *et al.*, 1993). The advantages of shared-care systems in general practice to medical management of illness in general have been reviewed by Orton (1994) but the need for careful planning is emphasised.

The benefits of the Glasgow system over 2 years were a reduced drop-out rate (3% versus 14%) and more adequate review of the patients compared to routine clinic follow-up (McInnes and McGhee, 1995). The shared-care system was also more cost-effective – £28.96 versus £50.55 per adequate review. In addition to the benefits for the patient, large shared care clinics offer opportunities for long-term observational research and audit.

In summary, the practical aims (10 commandments) when treating an elderly patient with raised blood pressure are:

1. Ensure sustained hypertension

2. Look at all cardiovascular risk factors
   - smoking
   - excessive alcohol
   - obesity
   - lipids etc.
3. Non-drug measures to lower blood pressure
   - optimise alcohol intake
   - weight reduction
   - reduce salt
   - potassium intake
4. Discuss risks with patient
5. Drug therapy if patient is willing
6. Select drug for individual patient
   - usually thiazide first
   - 50% need more than one drug
7. Decide on individual target blood pressure
8. Avoid overtreatment and adverse effects
9. Some reduction in blood pressure with well-tolerated drugs is better than none if the patient doesn't take medication because of the adverse effects
10. Adequate follow-up.

In conclusion, treating hypertension in elderly patients is a rewarding activity even though we do not see the instant benefits of therapy. Evidence-based medicine (at least partly) can be practised to achieve benefits for the patient, the providers of health care and the system of health care as a whole. Clearly there is still a need for further research in all aspects of hypertension from the underlying mechanisms through development and evaluation of new drugs to the most effective way to deliver care. There is a major challenge in achieving control of hypertension in elderly patients, many of whom have multiple problems that affect the choice of drug and response to treatment. Several important clinical trials will be published in the 2–3 years after publication of this volume. This reflects the growing interest in antihypertensive treatment for elderly patients and the excitement of working in an important area of preventative medicine. It is gratifying to know that future editions will contain information to enable practitioners to move closer to the ideal of evidence-based medicine.

REFERENCES

Ford GA, Duggan S, Aylett M, Eccles M 1996. Validation of primary care notes based hypertension audit tool. Presented to the British Geriatrics Society, April 1996. *Age and Ageing* **25**(2), 66.

Hannah J, Kennedy S, McGhee S, McInnes G 1993. Shared care: the way ahead for hypertension? *Prescriber* October, 19–23.

Haq IU, Jackson PR, Yeo WW, Ramsay LE 1995. Sheffield risk and treatment table for cholesterol lowering for primary prevention of coronary heart disease. *Lancet* **346**, 1467–71.

Holmen J, Forsen L, Hjort PF, Midthjell K, Waaler HT, Bjorndal A 1991. Detecting hypertension: screening versus case finding in Norway. *British Medical Journal* **302**, 219–22.

Hypertension Guidelines Committee 1991. *Hypertension diagnosis, treatment and maintenance*. Guidelines endorsed by the High Blood Pressure Research Council of Australia. Adelaide: Royal Australian College of General Practitioners.

Jackson R, Barham P, Bills J *et al.* 1993. Management of raised blood pressure in New Zealand: a discussion document. *British Medical Journal* **307**, 107–10.

Joint National Committee on Detection, Evaluation and Treatment of High Blood Pressure 1993. Fifth Report. *Archives of Internal Medicine* **153**, 154–83.

McInnes GT, McGhee SM 1995. Delivery of care for hypertension. *Journal of Human Hypertension* **9**, 429–33.

Orton P 1994. Shared care. *Lancet* **344**, 1413–15.

Petrie JC, Robb OJ, Webster J, Scott AK, Jeffers TA, Park MD 1985. Computer assisted shared care in hypertension. *British Medical Journal* **290**, 1960–2.

Sever P, Beevers G, Bulpitt C *et al.* 1993. Management guidelines in essential hypertension. Report of the second working party of the British Hypertension Society. *British Medical Journal* **306**, 983–7.

Swales JD 1995. The growth of medical science: the lessons of Malthus. *Journal of the Royal College of Physicians of London* **29**, 490–501.

Appendix

SHANGHAI TRIAL OF NIFEDIPINE IN THE ELDERLY (STONE)

In Chapters 4 and 5, reference was made to ongoing trials of newer antihypertensive agents. The only one which has reported to date (January 1997) is the STONE study (Gong *et al.*, 1996). This trial was begun in 1986 before the results of the large studies such as STOP-Hypertension and SHEP had reported. It was thus considered ethical to compare nifedipine, as the active treatment, with placebo. A single-blind design was used and the most severely affected patients on placebo were reallocated to active treatment. There was a 10% interchange between placebo and active groups which is lower than in SHEP or EWPHE. A total of 1632 patients aged 60–79 years were recruited.

There was a significant reduction in stroke from 36 events on long-acting nifedipine to 16 on placebo (relative risk: 0.43; 95% CI 0.24–0.77), and in total cardiovascular events from 59 to 23 (relative risk: 0.38; 95% CI 0.24–0.61). A major drawback from a Western viewpoint is the rarity of myocardial infarction in this population – only two events each in placebo and active treatment groups.

This trial has shown that nifedipine can reduce the risk of stroke in elderly patients with hypertension and is at least comparable to older agents such as thiazide diuretics. We need to await other trial results from populations with a greater risk of myocardial infarction to see if there is any extra benefit. At present, low dose thiazide diuretics should remain the drug of choice in older adults with hypertension. However, at least nifedipine can now be used with confidence in patients in whom thiazides and beta-blockers are ineffective or not tolerated.

REFERENCE

Gong L, Zhang W, Zhu Y *et al.*, 1996. Shanghai Trial of Nifedipine in the Elderly (STONE). *Journal of Hypertension* **14**, 1237–45.

Index

Accutracker II ambulatory monitor, 107
Acebutolol, 59, 82
Acetylcholine, 23
Adrenaline, 25
Adverse effects of antihypertensives, 4, 161, 178–81
  ACE inhibitors, 94–5
  alpha-blocking drugs, 97–8
  beta-blockers, 84–5
  calcium channel antagonists, 89–90
  centrally acting drugs, 79–80
  clinical trials, 46, 51, 54
  discussion with patient, 187–8
  loop diuretics, 74–5
  prediction, 188–9
  thiazide diuretics, 70–2
Age factors
  determinants of hypertension, 11, 13
  and distribution of blood pressure, 6–8
  nocturnal blood pressure, 115–16
Albuminuria, 27
Alcohol
  determinant of hypertension, 13, 132–3, 134, 143
  protection against cardiovascular disease, 13
  reduction, 189
Aldosterone, 26, 27
Aldosteronism, 71, 75, 76
Allopurinol, 72
Alpha-blocking drugs
  costs, 153
  pharmacology, 96–8
  and postural hypotension, 28
  psychomotor performance, 173
Alprenolol, 82
Ambulatory blood pressure measurement (ABPM), 3,
    103–5, 124, 186
  advantages and limitations, 9
  diagnosis and management of hypertension in the
    elderly, 109–21
  evaluation of new agents, 123
  left ventricular hypertrophy, 56
  normal population, 108–9
  selection and evaluation of antihypertensives, 122–3
  technical aspects, 106–8
Amiloride
  adverse effects, 71, 180
  clinical trials, 47, 50, 78
  pharmacology, 75, 76, 77
  psychomotor performance, 167, 171
Aminoglycosides, 75
Amlodipine, 59, 61, 87, 88, 89
Angina, 31
Angiotensin I, 22
Angiotensin II, 22, 26, 27
Angiotensin-converting enzyme inhibitors (ACE
    inhibitors)
  ambulatory blood pressure measurement, 123
  cardiovascular diseases, 57–8
  cost-effectiveness, 153, 156, 193

and dietary sodium restriction, 136
  diuretics, 27
  indications, 93, 187
  interactions with other drugs, 72, 73, 75, 77, 95–6
  left ventricular hypertrophy, 56
  pharmacology, 91–6
  psychomotor performance, 170, 172, 173
  quality of life, 177
  renal artery stenosis, 34
Antihypertensives, 63–4
  adverse effects, see Adverse effects of
    antihypertensives
  appropriateness, 186–7
  cardiovascular diseases, 57–8
  costs, 153–4, 156, 157, 158
  intermediate endpoints, 55
  isolated systolic hypertension, 10
  left ventricular hypertrophy, 30, 55–7
  major outcome studies, 40–55
  new drugs, 63
  peripheral resistance reduction, 22
  pharmacology, see Pharmacology of
    antihypertensives
  requirements, 188–9
  selection and evaluation, 122–3
  versus non-pharmacological management, 141–3
Arterial wall rigidity, 9, 22–4, 26
Arteriolar constriction, mechanisms affecting, 22–4
Arteriosclerosis, 32
Association for the Advancement of Medical
    Instrumentation (AAMI), 106, 108
Atenolol
  adverse effects, 46, 51, 179, 180, 181
  clinical trials, 44, 45, 46, 47, 50, 52, 60
  comparisons with other antihypertensives, 61
  left ventricular hypertrophy, 56
  pharmacology, 81, 82, 83, 84
  psychomotor performance, 164, 165, 166, 167
  quality of life, 168, 169, 175, 176, 177
  versus non-pharmacological management, 141, 142
Atheroma, 29, 30, 31, 34
Atherosclerosis, 34
Atrial natriuretic peptide (ANP), 24, 26
Auscultatory gap, 9, 103–4
Australian therapeutic trial in mild hypertension, 40–1,
    43, 49, 54
Autonomic nervous system, 24
AV nipping, 31
Azapropazone, 72

Baroceptor control, 28–9
Baroreflex sensitivity, 110
Bendrofluazide
  clinical trials, 44, 45
  cost-effectiveness, 193
  left ventricular hypertrophy, 56–7
  pharmacology, 69, 70, 71, 73
  quality of life, 168, 175

Benzodiazepines, 172
Beta-blockers
  adverse effects, 54, 84–5, 161, 179, 180, 181
  ambulatory blood pressure measurement, 123
  clinical trials, 47, 51, 86
  contraindications, 60, 84
  cost-effectiveness, 153, 156, 157, 158
  and dietary sodium restriction, 136
  effectiveness, 186
  guidelines, 191
  interactions with other drugs, 72, 73, 80, 85–6, 90
  left ventricular hypertrophy, 56
  pharmacology, 81–6
  psychomotor performance, 165, 166, 170, 171–2
  quality of life, 175–7
  stroke, 61
Beta-sympathomimetics, 75
Biofeedback, 140
Birth weight, 10
Bisoprolol, 82, 169, 177
Blood pressure, definition, 21–2
Body-mass index (BMI), 11–13, 17
  postural orthostatic hypotension, 10, 105
Borderline hypertension, 121
Bradykinin, 24
Branded drugs, costs, 153
British Hypertension Society (BHS), 106, 107, 108, 191, 192
Bumetanide, 73, 74

Calcium, 137–8
Calcium channel blockers
  adverse effects, 4, 89–90
  ambulatory blood pressure measurement, 123
  appropriateness, 186–7
  cardiovascular diseases, 57, 58
  comparisons, 61
  cost-effectiveness, 153, 156
Calcium channel blockers – *contd*
  falls, 62
  left ventricular hypertrophy, 56
  pharmacology, 86–91
  psychomotor performance, 172–3
  quality of life, 177
Captopril
  cardiovascular diseases, 57–8
  clinical trials, 55, 60
  comparisons with other antihypertensives, 61
  cost-effectiveness, 156, 193
  left ventricular hypertrophy, 56–7
  pharmacology, 92, 93, 94
  psychomotor performance, 165, 166, 172, 173
  quality of life, 169, 177
Cardiac complications, 29–30, 34
Cardiac failure, 57, 69, 70
Cardiac muscle, 26
Cardiac output, 25–6
Cardiovascular disease (CVD), 2, 13–17, 46
Carotid artery stenosis, 10, 30
Carotid body, 28
Catecholamines, 24, 28, 86
Celiprolol, 82
Centrally acting drugs, 78–81, 166
Cephalosporins, 75
Cerebrovascular complications, 30–1, 34
Cerebrovascular disease (CVD), 154
CH-Druch sphygmomanometer, 108

Chlorothiazide, 40, 73
Chlorthalidone, 73
  adverse effects, 179
  clinical trials, 52, 59
  pharmacokinetics, 69
  psychomotor performance, 164, 170
  quality of life, 168, 174, 176
  versus non-pharmacological management, 142
Cholesterol, 28, 29, 71
Chronic vascular disease (CVD), 15
Cilazapril, 93
Claudication, 31
Clonidine
  clinical trials, 60, 81
  pharmacology, 78, 79, 80
  psychomotor performance, 173
Coamilozide, 164, 169
Cognitive function, 163
Combined dietary supplements, 138–9
Co-morbidity, 14–15
Complications of hypertension, 29–34
Continuation of therapy, 62
Continuous ambulatory blood pressure monitoring, 110
Coope and Warrender trial, 43, 44–7, 49, 54, 175–6
Coronary arteries, 30
Coronary heart disease (CHD), 14, 17, 71, 154
Coronary reserve, 28
Corticosteroids, 72, 75
Cost analysis (cost-minimisation analysis, CMA), 149–50, 157
Cost-benefit analysis, 149, 150, 157
Cost-effectiveness of treatments, 3–4, 148–9, 158–9, 192–3
  costs and benefits of treatments, 153–5, 190
  methods for establishing, 149–52
  review, 155–7
Cost-utility analysis (CUA), 149, 150, 155, 156
Cotton-wool spots, 32
Creatinine, 44
Cyclopenthiazide, 69, 73
Cyclosporin, 90

Daytime blood pressure, 56, 109, 110
Diabetes, 70, 72, 77
Diagnosis of hypertension, 3, 109–21, 186
Dietary supplements, 138–9
Digoxin, 72, 75, 77, 90
Dihydropyridines, 87, 88, 89, 91
  adverse effects, 4, 89, 90
  interactions with other drugs, 85, 86, 90
Diltiazem
  cardiovascular diseases, 58
  clinical trials, 60, 90
  comparisons with other hypertensives, 61
  pharmacology, 85, 87, 88, 89, 90
  psychomotor performance, 166, 171, 172, 173
  quality of life, 169, 176, 177
Dippers, 115, 116, 117, 121
Disopyramide, 85
Diuretics (*see also* loop diuretics; potassium-sparing diuretics; thiazide diuretics)
  adverse effects, 180, 181
  ambulatory blood pressure measurement, 123
  clinical trials, 42, 44, 46, 47, 50, 51
  cost-effectiveness, 153, 156, 157, 158
  guidelines, 191
  interactions with other drugs, 95

Diuretics – *contd*
  left ventricular hypertrophy, 56
  psychomotor performance, 165, 166, 167–71
  quality of life, 174–5, 177
  renin-angiotensin-aldosterone system, 27
  toleration, 64
Dosing boxes, 189
Doxazosin, 59, 96, 173
Dyspepsia, 31

Echocardiography (ECG)
  abnormalities, 10, 17
  ambulatory blood pressure measurement, 119
  left ventricular hypertrophy, 55, 56, 57
Elastic fibres, 23
Elderly, definition, 2
Enalapril
  cardiovascular diseases, 57
  clinical trials, 55, 59, 97
  comparisons with other antihypertensives, 61
  cost-effectiveness, 193
  pharmacology, 92, 93
  psychomotor performance, 165, 166, 170, 171, 172, 173
  quality of life, 169, 176, 177
Endothelial factors, arteriolar constriction, 22–3
Endothelin-1, 22
Environmental factors, 10, 11
Ethanol, 13
European Working Party on High blood pressure in the Elderly trial (EWPHE), 41–4, 49, 54, 175, 178
Exercise, 13, 140, 189
Exudates, 32

Fats, dietary, 139–40
Felodipine, 87, 89
Fish oils, 139
Flecainide, 85
Focal retinal ischaemia, 32
Foetal environment, 10
Follow-up procedures, 194
Fosinopril, 93
Framingham study, 43, 163
Frusemide, 73, 74

Gender factors
  beta-blockers, 84
  body weight, 28
  distribution of blood pressure, 6–8
  isolated systolic hypertension, 9
  prevalence of hypertension, 8–9
General practitioner consultations, 153–4
Generic drugs, costs, 153
Genetic factors, 10, 25
Glaucoma, 32
Glomerular filtration, 26
Glomerular function, loss of, 33
Guidelines on hypertension management, 191–2
Gull, William Withey, 1

Haemorrhagic stroke, 30, 31
Hales, Stephen, 1, 110
Hard exudates, 32
Harvey, William, 1
Hawksley random zero sphygmomanometer, 106
Heart attack, 23
Heart rate, 25, 110–11

High pressure glaucoma, 32
Hyaline change, 33
Hydralazine, 97
  cost-effectiveness, 155
  interactions with other drugs, 85
  psychomotor performance, 170
  quality of life, 168, 176
Hydrochlorothiazide
  adverse effects, 70–1, 178, 180
  clinical trials, 42, 47, 50, 60
  comparisons with other antihypertensives, 61
  cost-effectiveness, 155, 156
  pharmacology, 69, 70–1, 73, 77
  psychomotor performance, 165, 167, 170, 171
  quality of life, 168, 169, 175, 176
Hydroflumethazide, 73
Hypertension, definition, 2, 8, 184–5
Hypertension Stroke Co-operative Study Group (HSCS), 54
Hypotension, 105, 116–17
  postural, *see* Postural orthostatic hypotension

Inappropriate hypertension, 105
Indoramin, 96
Information leaflets, 187
Insulin, 28, 71
Intellectual function, 163
Ischaemic heart disease, 29, 30, 46, 188
Ischaemic stroke, 30
Isolated systolic hypertension (ISH)
  ambulatory blood pressure measurement, 106
  auscultatory gap, 104
  comparisons of antihypertensives, 61
  major outcome studies, 51, 52–3
  nocturnal blood pressure, 116, 117–20
  postural hypotension, 104
  prevalence, 9–10
  psychomotor performance, 167
  very elderly people, 63
Isosorbide, 97
Isradipine, 61, 87, 89
  quality of life, 169, 176, 177

Japanese trial, 54

Kinins, 23–4
Korotkov sounds, 104

Labetolol, 82
Lacidipine, 87, 89
Left ventricular hypertrophy (LVH), 29, 30
  arteriolar constriction, 23
  assessment, 25–6
  effects of treatment, 55–7
  nocturnal blood pressure, 115, 116
Leg oedema, 4
Levodopa, 80
Lifestyle changes, *see* Non-pharmacological management
Lignocaine, 85
Lipids, 71, 96
Lisinopril, 58, 93
Lithium, 72, 77, 90
Loop diuretics
  indications, 70, 74, 187
  pharmacology, 73–5, 77
  renal artery stenosis, 34
Losartan, 63

Magnesium, 138–9
Malignant hypertension, 33–4
Meals, effects on blood pressure, 9, 105
Mean, regression to the, 9, 25
Measurement of blood pressure, 3, 9, 103–5, 191 (*see also* Ambulatory blood pressure measurement)
Medical Research Council (MRC) hypertension trial, 43, 49–51, 54, 181
Meditation, 189
Men, *see* Gender factors
Menopause, 6, 28
Mercury sphygmomanometer, 106, 107
Meta-analysis of outcome trials, 53–5
Methyldopa
    adverse effects, 79, 178
    clinical trials, 42, 44, 80–1
    pharmacology, 78–9, 80
    psychomotor performance, 162, 165, 170, 173–4
    quality of life, 168, 175–6, 177
Metoprolol, 47, 82, 168, 176, 180
    psychomotor performance, 166, 170, 171, 172
Microalbuminuria, 27
Minoxidil, 74, 85
Moxonidine, 78
Myocardial infarction
    clinical trials, 43, 57–8
    costs, 154
    hypertension as risk factor, 17
    left ventricular function, 26, 30
    prevalence, 2, 31

Nadolol, 82
Neurogenic effects, 24
New drugs, 63
Nicardipine, 87, 89
Nifedipine
    adverse effects, 161
    cardiovascular diseases, 58
    clinical trials, 44, 50, 55, 91
    comparisons with other antihypertensives, 61
    cost-effectiveness, 156
    pharmacology, 87, 88, 89
    psychomotor performance, 165, 166, 171, 172, 173
    quality of life, 169, 177
Night-time blood pressure
    ambulatory blood pressure measurement, 115–16, 117
    left ventricular hypertrophy, 56
    variability, 109, 110
Nimodipine, 87
Nisoldipine, 87
Nitrendipine, 87, 91
Nitric oxide (NO), 23
Nocturnal blood pressure, *see* Night-time blood pressure
Non-dippers, 115, 116
Non-pharmacological management, 3, 129–30, 143–4
    alcohol, 132–3
    calcium, 137–8
    combined dietary supplements, 138–9
    cost-effectiveness, 154, 157, 158, 193
    dietary fats, 139
    dietary sodium, 133–6
    exercise and other behavioural methods, 140–1
    magnesium, 138
    potassium, 136–7
    requirements, 189
    vegetarian diet, 139

versus drug therapy, 141–3
    weight reduction, 130–2
Non-steroidal anti-inflammatory drugs (NSAIDs), 72, 75, 86, 95
Noradrenaline, 24, 28
Nottingham Health Profile (NHP), 174

Obesity, 11–13, 27–9, 120, 130
Oedema, leg, 4
Once-daily dosing, 189
Orthostatic hypotension, *see* Postural orthostatic hypotension
Osler's manoeuvre, 104
Osteoporosis, 140
Oxprenolol, 82, 85

Papilloedema, 32
Patent protection, 153
Patient information leaflets, 187
Penbutolol, 82
Perindopril, 92, 93
Peripheral resistance, 22–4, 26
Peripheral vascular disease, 29
Pharmacology of antihypertensives, 68
    ACE inhibitors, 91–6
    alpha-blocking drugs, 96–8
    beta-blockers, 81–6
    calcium channel antagonists, 86–91
    centrally acting drugs, 78–81
    loop diuretics, 73–5
    potassium-sparing diuretics, 75–8
    thiazide diuretics, 68–73
Phenothiazines, 80
Pindolol, 47, 82, 85, 180
Placental weight to birth weight ratio, 10
Polythiazide, 73
Portapres finger monitoring device, 110
Post-prandial falls in blood pressure, 9, 105
Postural orthostatic hypotension, 105
    ambulatory blood pressure measurement, 121
    baroceptor control, 28
    prevalence, 10
Potassium, 70–1, 136–7, 138–9
Potassium-sparing diuretics, 70, 71, 75–8, 96
Practolol, 82
Prazosin, 60, 96, 97, 156, 173
Pregnancy, 28
Prevalence of hypertension in elderly people, 8–10
Probenecid, 72
Propranolol, 81, 82, 83, 84, 156
    psychomotor performance, 165, 170, 171–2
    quality of life, 169, 176–7
Prostatism, 97, 98
Pseudohypertension, 104, 105
Pseudohypotension, 104
Psychomotor performance (PP), 161–3, 164–6, 173–4
    ACE inhibitors, 173
    beta-blockers, 171–2
    calcium channel blockers, 172–3
    diuretics, 167–71
    studies not controlling for drug class, 163–7

Quality adjusted life year (QALY), 150
Quality of life (QOL), 161–2, 168–9, 174, 177–8
    ACE inhibitors, 177
    beta-blockers, 175–7
    calcium channel blockers, 177

Quality of life (QOL) – *contd*
  diuretics, 174–5
  importance, 4
Quinapril, 93

Race, 60, 84
Ramipril, 58, 93, 193
Raynaud's phenomenon, 89, 97
Reflex control, 28–9
Regression dilution bias, 11
Regression to the mean, 9, 25
Relaxation, 140, 189
Renal artery stenosis, 34
Renal disease, 27, 32, 34
Renal failure, 26
Renal function, 27, 32–4
Renal stone disease, 70
Renal tubules, 24
Renin-angiotensin-aldosterone system, 26, 27
Renovascular disease, 32, 93, 95
Reserpine
  adverse effects, 179
  cost-effectiveness, 155
  psychomotor performance, 164, 170, 173
  quality of life, 168, 176
Resistance vessels, structural change in, 22, 24
Retinal complications, 31–2
Retinal ischaemia, 32
Retinal vein occlusion, 32
Rilmenidine, 78
Rule of halves, 45, 64, 192

Salbutamol, 72, 86
Screening, 64, 185
Seasonal variation in blood pressure, 9
Shared-care schemes, 70, 194
Sickness Impact Profile (SIP), 174
Sick sinus syndrome, 85
Side effects, *see* Adverse effects of antihypertensives
Silver wiring, 31
Single drug therapy for hypertension in men study,
  60–1
Smoking, 29, 51, 84, 86, 189
Smooth muscle, 23, 24
Sodium
  determinant of hypertension, 11, 28, 133–6, 143
  load, 26–7
  and potassium, interaction between, 136–7
Sotalol, 82
SpaceLabs 90202 sphygmomanometer, 106
SpaceLabs 90207 sphygmomanometer, 108
Spironolactone, 75, 76, 77, 78
Stepped care regimes, 155, 156, 158
Stress, 24–5
Stroke, 30–1
  antihypertensives, effects, 188
  arteriolar constriction, 23
  atheroma, 29
  clinical trials, 43, 46–7, 48
  cost-effectiveness of hypertension treatment, 154
  hypertension as risk factor, 14
  prevalence, 2
Stroke volume, 25–6
Sulphonamides, 74
Sulphonylureas, 72
Sustained hypertension, 3, 9, 27
Sustained isolated systolic hypertension, 118, 119

Swedish trial in old patients with hypertension (STOP-
  Hypertension), 43, 47–9, 54, 157, 180
Sympathetic nervous system, 28
Syndrome X, 28
Systolic Hypertension in the Elderly Program (SHEP),
  10, 43, 49, 52–3, 179
  quality of life, 174–5, 176

Terbutaline, 72, 86
Terazosin, 96
Theophylline, 90
Thiazide diuretics
  adverse effects, 54, 70–2, 161, 179, 181
  clinical trials, 46, 47, 53, 73
  comparisons with other antihypertensives, 61
  cost-effectiveness, 193
  effectiveness, 186
  guidelines, 191–2
  individual characteristics, 73
  interactions with other drugs, 72, 75, 77, 80
  pharmacology, 68–70
  quality of life, 175
  stroke, 60–1
  tolerance, 64
Thrombotic stroke, 30
Timolol, 82, 84
Tracking, blood pressure, 10, 13
Trandolapril, 93
Transient ischaemic attack, 30, 31
Transient isolated systolic hypertension, 118, 120
Treatment of Mild Hypertension study (TOMHS), 59–60
Triamterene
  adverse effects, 70–1, 178
  clinical trials, 42, 78
  comparisons with other antihypertensives, 61
  pharmacology, 75, 76, 77
  psychomotor performance, 165
  quality of life, 175

Urea, 71
Uricosuric drugs, 72

Variability of blood pressure, 9, 103, 110–11
Vascular disease, risk, 190
Vascular smooth muscle, 23, 24
Vasodilators, 23
Vegetarian diet, 139
Verapamil
  cardiovascular disease, 58
  comparisons with other antihypertensives, 61
  left ventricular hypertrophy, 56
  pharmacology, 85, 87, 88, 89, 90, 91
Veterans Administration Study Group (VACS), 54

Warrender, T.S., *see* Coope and Warrender trial
Weight, *see* Body-mass index
Weight reduction, 130–2, 143, 189
White-coat effect, 112, 113
White-coat hypertension
  ambulatory blood pressure measurement, 111–15, 121,
    122
  diagnosis, 186
  heart rate, 25
  and measurement problems, 9
  minimisation, 189–90
Withey Gull, William, 1
Women, *see* Gender factors